Healthy Hair

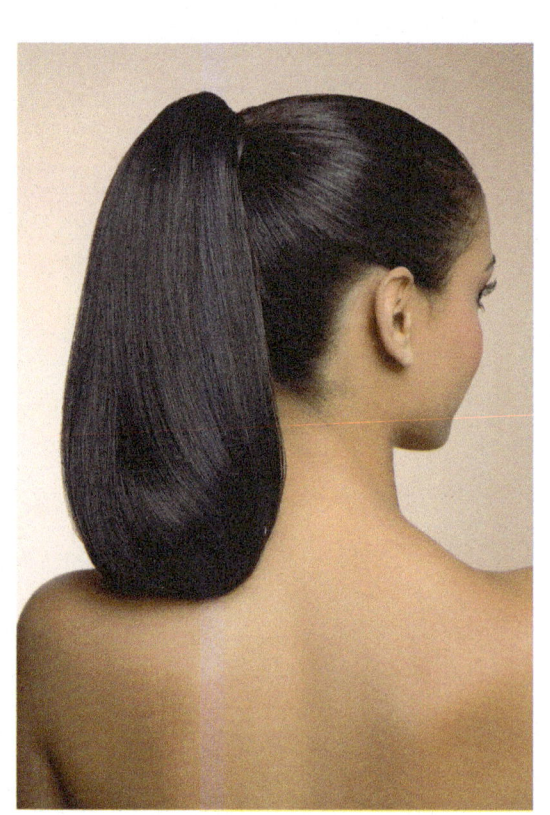

Jennifer Marsh · John Gray
Antonella Tosti

Healthy Hair

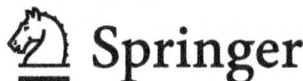

Jennifer Marsh
The Procter & Gamble Company
Mason, OH, USA

John Gray
Winston Park, Gillitts, South Africa

Antonella Tosti
Department of Dermatology and
    Cutaneous Surgery
University of Miami Leonard M. Miller
    School of Medicine
Miami, FL, USA

ISBN 978-3-319-34916-9   ISBN 978-3-319-18386-2   (eBook)
DOI 10.1007/978-3-319-18386-2

Springer Cham Heidelberg New York Dordrecht London
© Springer International Publishing Switzerland 2015
Softcover reprint of the hardcover 1st edition 2015
This work is subject to copyright. All rights are reserved by the Publisher, whether the whole or part of the material is concerned, specifically the rights of translation, reprinting, reuse of illustrations, recitation, broadcasting, reproduction on microfilms or in any other physical way, and transmission or information storage and retrieval, electronic adaptation, computer software, or by similar or dissimilar methodology now known or hereafter developed.
The use of general descriptive names, registered names, trademarks, service marks, etc. in this publication does not imply, even in the absence of a specific statement, that such names are exempt from the relevant protective laws and regulations and therefore free for general use.
The publisher, the authors and the editors are safe to assume that the advice and information in this book are believed to be true and accurate at the date of publication. Neither the publisher nor the authors or the editors give a warranty, express or implied, with respect to the material contained herein or for any errors or omissions that may have been made.

Printed on acid-free paper

Springer International Publishing AG Switzerland is part of Springer Science+Business Media (www.springer.com)

Foreword

Beware of her fair hair, for she excels all women in the magic of her locks; And when she winds them round a young man's neck, She will not ever set him free again.

—Goethe

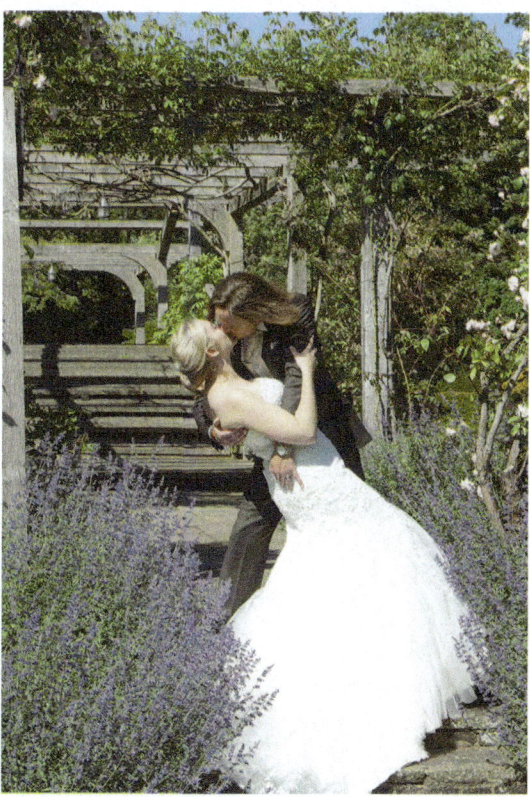

Fig. 1 More time and effort is spent on the bride's hair than perhaps on any other day of her life. Healthy hair sends a powerful message of youth and health. In this case—from both parties

Hair is one of nature's survivors and although technically 'dead', one of the most resilient. The visible hair shaft appears very simple, but the mechanism to create it, the hair follicle deep in the skin, is one of the most complex biological systems nature has devised.

Hair first arrived on the evolutionary scene some 310 million years ago on reptilian-like animals. It preceded and survived the rise and extinction of the dinosaurs and emerged as the dominant skin appendage of mammals. As part of this class, modern humans have 'inherited' skin which although bearing several million hair follicles have largely confined growing hair to the scalp.

Caring for hair is entirely consistent with mammalian grooming which enhances appearance and subconsciously imparts status, health, physical attractiveness and, perhaps less romantically, helps remove parasites. Hair care is an (almost) ubiquitous human habit in the twenty-first century and is driven by conscious as well as subconscious social and evolutionary pressures.

The varied appearance of human hair type can be explained by genetic inheritance (genotype) in association with adaptive consequences to the environment and sexual selection that occurred after modern humans spread out from their origins in Africa some 70–90,000 years ago. These differences now play an important role in determining grooming habits and the type of hair-care products women use as part of their grooming ritual.

Why then a book devoted to the topic of 'healthy hair' and hair-care cosmetics?

In an age of celebrity where the outward manifestation, be it conforming or renegade, is ever more socially important in most human societies, the health and hence appearance of scalp hair should be of importance. Research [1] illustrates the importance of the symbiosis of healthy hair framing a healthy face. However, self-inflicted damage to hair through a constant desire to improve or change nature has led to an unprecedented epidemic of cosmetic hair damage and is THE most common hair issue to affect women.

Improving the understanding of the causes of hair damage and assisting in the correct selection and application of cosmetic hair-care products are our mission. It is to the dispersal of this knowledge we devote this publication with the earnest hope that it will touch lives and improve quality of life for millions of women.

Reference

1. Gray, J. International Congress & Symposium Series 266_Assessment of hair quality using eye-tracking technology. London: RSM Press. 2006.

Mason, OH, USA	Jennifer Marsh
Winston Park, Gillitts, South Africa	John Gray
Miami, FL, USA	Antonella Tosti

Acknowledgements

The author "Jennifer Marsh" would like to acknowledge my coauthors of the book, Dr John Gray and Antonella Tosti, for their tremendous support and also for making the process a fun one. Also thanks to Procter & Gamble for allowing me to follow my passions for fundamental science and understanding hair health and bring that experience to the readers of this book. Finally, to my husband for always being there every step of the way.

The author "John Gray" would like to acknowledge coauthors Professor Antonella Tosti for her tremendous knowledge, energy, and unflagging support over many years. Dr Jennifer Marsh for her unsurpassed technical expertise in all things relating to the hair shaft and hair care technologies. The remarkable Research and Development scientists of Procter & Gamble for their inestimable support and advice and the members of the Pantene Hair Research Institute for their inspiration to attempt this publication.

To Glynis Richards. Stylist in Durban, South Africa, for sharing her tremendous talent and knowledge and her help in developing practical advice in styling.

Tina Beckbessinger one of our two guinea pig models: an example of willpower and triumph over a life-threatening condition requiring a heart/lung transplant.

To my long suffering and dear wife for her love, support, and participation as our other guinea pig model.

Finally, to all those ladies on the streets of the world whose photographs populate this publication in the hope that it will bring understanding of the route to HEALTHY HAIR.

The author "Antonella Tosti" is so happy to have been involved in this project! Thanks Jennifer and John, it was so interesting to share a project with scientists with a common interest but a different approach and knowledge. Thanks to my husband Luca and my children Lorenzo e Margherita who always support me.

Contents

1 Healthy Hair: Form and Function 1
  Hair 1
    Human Hair and the Follicle 1
    The Hair Cycle 5
  Hair: The Cosmetic Aspects 11
    The Terminal Hair Shaft 11
    The Cuticle 12
    The Cortex 13
    The Medulla 14
    Abnormal Hairs 14
    Hair Diameter and Texture 15
    Hair Types 15
    Phenotype and "Hair Health" 15
    Classification of Hair Phenotypes 16
    Sub-Equatorial African Hair 16
    Australasian Hair 17
    East Asian Straight Hair 17
    Indo-European/Continental European Hair 19
    Hair Phenotypes in the Americas 20
    Developments of Human Hair Differences 20
    Evolutionary Advantages of Straight and Curly Hair 21
    Hair Color 21
    Gray Hair 22
    The Physical Properties of Hair 22
    Porosity 22
    Elasticity 24
    Static Electricity 24
    Texture 25
  Reference 28
  Further Reading 28

2 Root-to-Tip Hair Health 29
  Introduction 29
  Healthy Hair 29
    Women's Perception of Hair Health 30
    Sign 1: Shine 32
    Shine Summary 37

Sign 2: Absence of Split Ends/Damaged Tips	37
Sign 3: Smoothness/Frizz-Free	40
Sign 4: Volume	42
Sign 5: No Breakage/Strength	43
References	44

3 Understanding Hair Damage 45

Introduction: The Hair Mass	45
Hair in Time and Space	45
The Process of 'Weathering'	46
Sources of Damage	46
The Record of the Hair	46
Causes of Hair Damage	47
Hair Damage: Women's Perspective	50
Women's Perception of Causes of Damage	50
Global Perspective	51
Summary	52
Psychological Consequences of Unhealthy Hair	52
Bad Hair Day Study	52
Hair and Face as Social Signals	52
Experimental Evidence of Root-to-Tip Hair Damage	55
Damage Insults	56
Specific Forms of Damage	58
Physical Processes	60
Environmental Processes	61
Heat Processes	63
Chemical Treatments	66
Minimising Damage	70
General Principles	70
References	70

4 Healthy Hair Method Assessments 71

Introduction	71
Multiple Strategies to Assess Hair Health	73
Strategy 1: Assessment of Hair (Self or Observer)	74
Strategy 2: Single Fibre Mechanical Properties	80
Strategy 3: Structural Property Measures	82
Summary	84
References	84

5 Clinical Signs of Hair Damage 85

Introduction	85
Symptoms of Hair Damage	85
Hair Breakage	86
Clinical Presentation Depending on Causes	87
Clinical Presentation Depending on Ethnicity	87
Diagnosis	91
Hair Knotting, Tangling, and Matting	92
Changes in the Hair Colour	94
References	94

6 Hair Density Reduction ... 97
Introduction ... 97
Acute Telogen Effluvium ... 97
Chronic Telogen Effluvium ... 97
Diffuse Alopecia ... 98
    Anagen Effluvium ... 98
    Patterned Alopecia (Androgenetic Alopecia) ... 98
    Alopecia Areata ... 99
References ... 99

7 Cosmetic Products and Hair Health ... 101
Introduction ... 101
The History of Hair Care and Hair-Care Products ... 101
Hair-Care Regimens ... 103
    History of Regimens for Different Hair Types ... 103
Hair-Care Products for Different Hair Needs ... 105
    Shampoos ... 105
    Modern Shampoo Formulations ... 106
    Key Ingredients of Shampoos ... 107
    Conditioners ... 110
    Conditioning Products in Ethnic Usage ... 111
    Oil Inclusion in Conditioning Products ... 112
    Key Ingredients of Conditioners ... 112
    Ethnic and Cultural Differences in Conditioning Preferences ... 112
    How to Select the Correct Hair-Care Regimen ... 113
Practical Aspects of Hair Care ... 117
    Cleansing (Shampooing) ... 117
Step by Step: Shampooing ... 118
    General Tips ... 119
Step by Step: Conditioning ... 119
    General Tips ... 121
    Summary ... 121
Styling and Hair Health ... 123
    Styling Problems ... 124
Styling Products ... 127
    Hairspray ... 128
    Mousse ... 129
    Hair Gels/Waxes/Pomades ... 129
Tips for Healthy Styling ... 129

Index ... 133

Abbreviations

BKT	Brazilian keratin treatments
EMG	Electron micrograph
HMI	Hair mass index
KAPs	Keratin-associated proteins
RH	Relative humidity
ROS	Reactive oxygen species
SEM	Scanning electron microscope
TAS	Terminal amino silicones
TEM	Transmission electron microscopy

About the Authors

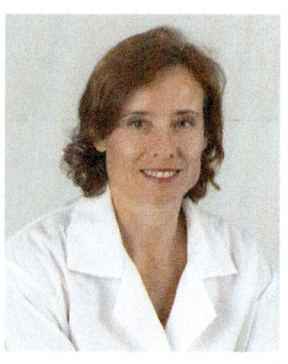

Dr Jennifer Marsh has a chemistry degree and Ph.D. from the University of Oxford and 2 years post-doc experience at Texas A&M University in the area of synthetic inorganic chemistry.

She has worked for the Procter & Gamble Company for 20 years in both hair care and hair color. During that time, she has worked in many different areas including new methods for measuring hair damage, developing new oxidants for hair colorants, and identifying chelants as a strategy for reducing hair damage. She has published numerous journal articles as well as presented her work at the major hair and cosmetic conferences. She is also a member of the Pantene Hair Research Institute.

Her current position is Research Fellow in the Beauty Technology Division where she leads technology development for P&G's hair care brands including Pantene. She lives in Cincinnati where she enjoys her passion for hair and technology development as well as playing squash and mountain biking.

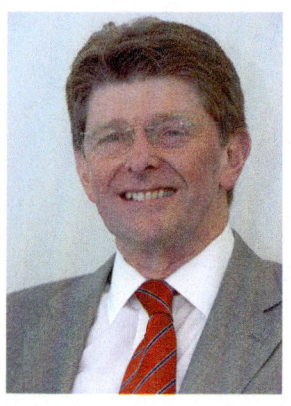

Dr John Gray trained in medicine at St Georges Medical School, London, and entered family practice where he developed his interest in dermatology and particularly hair disorders including opening a Hair Treatment Clinic.

In addition, he is the Medical Advisor to Procter & Gamble and has 30 years experience in their hair and skin care division. He has acted as Chair of many Premier Science Panel round table discussions with external experts relating to hair and skin care initiatives, and from 1997 to 2005, he was a Director of the Oxford Hair Foundation.

During this time, he published many textbooks, chapters, and pamphlets on hair and hair care cosmetics including the World of Hair and the Royal Society of Medicine Congress series.

He is an elected member of the European Academy of Dermatology and, the European and North American Hair Research Societies and was raised to be a Fellow of the Institute of Trichologists in 2013.

He now lives in Durban, South Africa, and pursues his fascination with photographing and understanding hair and hair care habits and practices in a vibrant multicultural society.

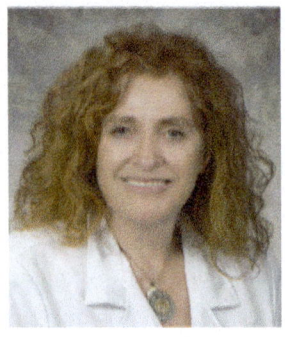

Dr Antonella Tosti is an Italian physician and scientist who is a worldwide recognized expert in hair and nail disorders.

She is a founding member and past president of the European Hair Research Society and member of Board of Directors of the North American Research Society.

She is the author of *Dermoscopy of Hair and Scalp Disorders*, the first hair and scalp dermoscopy atlas ever published. A new completely revised edition of this book is now in the printing process. She is editor of four textbooks on diagnosis and treatment of Hair Disorders and three textbooks on Nail Disorders.

She is member of numerous dermatological societies including the American Academy of Dermatology, the American Dermatological Association, The North American Hair Research Society, the Women Dermatological Society, the North American Society for Contact Dermatitis, the European Hair Research Society, and the International Society of Dermatology.

Professor Antonella Tosti is author of over 650 scientific publications.

She is Professor of Dermatology at the University of Miami, Florida.

Healthy Hair: Form and Function

Hair

Hair in "good health" is of critical importance to many mammals, all of whom possess skin studied with hair follicles. The arctic survival properties imbued by the pelt of the polar bear and the camouflage afforded to the African Springbok bear testimony to this.

Humans belong to an only recently evolved group of mammals—the primates. Of the hair of our extinct hominid ancestors who bestrode the planet some 4–6 million years ago we can but surmise. "Modern" humans (homo sapiens) evolved in East-Africa as recently as 200–250,000 years ago. Today's six billion plus humans all evolved from a common female ancestor (African Eve) who lived about 120,000 years ago. No evidence of the nature (phenotype) of her hair is known but the science of genetics has enabled us to peer back into the past and make some assumptions about the evolution of human hair and its role in today's world.

Compared to our immediate relatives, the great apes, we appear, mistakenly, almost hairless. In reality human skin carries 2–5 million hair follicles but as a species we have adapted to our environment by concentrating hair growth primarily to selected areas. The head is the most important but as part of our evolutionary path we still bear visible hair in areas associated with scenting and reproduction (Fig. 1.1).

Many mammals invest 30 % of their dietary protein in the manufacture of hair. Humans invest extraordinary amounts of protein even at a young age in growing scalp hair to a greater length than any other mammal. Sadly, failure to care for this precious commodity can place an individual outside of the common "herd" (Figs. 1.2 and 1.3).

The length of an individual's hair depends on the duration of continuous growth (anagen). Only the merino sheep has a comparable duration, although this is artificially induced by selective breeding.

It is open to debate quite why Homo sapiens is so blessed with profuse head hair when young and why subsequently so many lose it (Fig. 1.4).

Human hair's function may be that of a critical signaling device, conveying both age and health and even social status to others of the species. In prime condition it can act as a powerful beacon of sexual attraction: in a damaged or disheveled state—quite the reverse.

It is deep in the skin that the mysteries of hair begin—within the hair follicle.

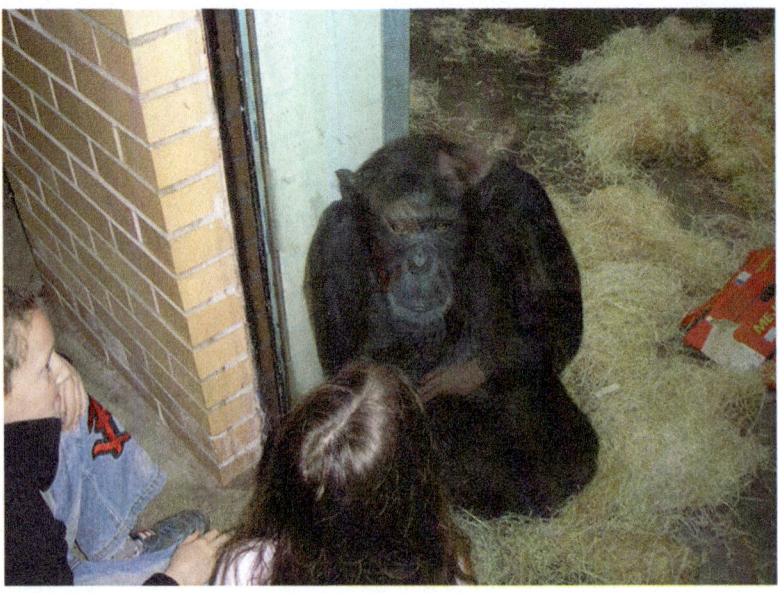

Fig. 1.1 Pan troglodytes (Chimpanzee) and young of the Homo sapiens species. Body hair in good condition is important to the former: scalp hair to the latter

Human Hair and the Follicle

This publication focuses primarily on the hair shaft. However, consideration of where the visible hair originates and what influence the follicle has on hair health is not unimportant.

The Hair Follicle

By definition a follicle is a mammalian skin organ that produces hair. It contains many of the complex biological systems found throughout the body and is a reservoir of stem cells which can produce either hairs or skin. These attributes infer the fundamental importance of such tiny organs to the body as a whole and reflect our mammalian heritage where fur and pelts are essential to survival.

Of the 2–5 million hair follicles on the human body, those on the scalp are the most fascinating and important in our lives. Possibly as a mark of its importance, the hair follicle has, like the eye, brain, and male human reproductive organs, been granted "immune privilege" wherein it is protected from attack by our own immune system. It is believed that when this privilege breaks down, the condition alopecia areata can develop (see Chap. 6).

Types of Follicle

In infancy, hair follicles over the body are generally small although those on the scalp produce significant hairs.

After puberty and under the influence of sex hormones, selected follicles enlarge and develop sebaceous glands and terminal hairs are produced on other body areas, although there are large inter and extra regional differences. These large and heavily pigmented hairs are described as **terminal** hairs.

Of the 100,000–150,000 scalp follicles, between 75 and 90 % produce terminal hairs. The associated sebaceous glands deliver sebum—a natural mixture of triglycerides, wax esters, and squalene. This helps to maintain the integrity of the scalp and has both protective and thermoregulatory properties.

Hair

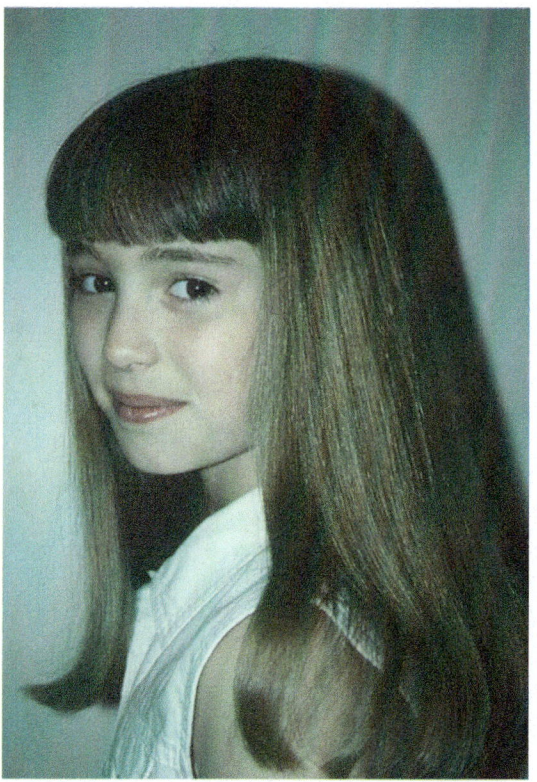

Fig. 1.2 Female aged, 7 massive amounts of protein to manufacture a signaling device of youth and health

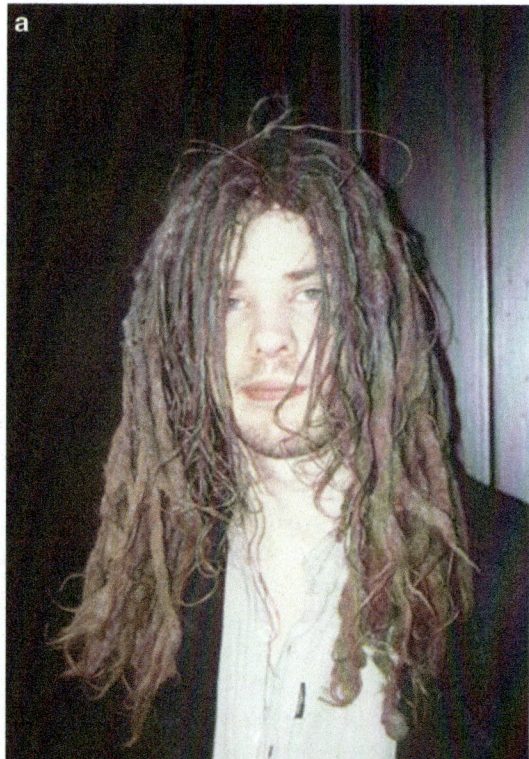

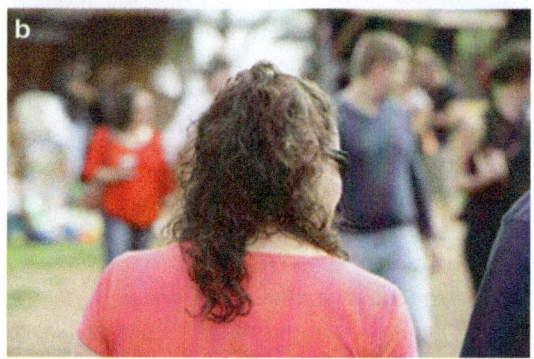

Fig. 1.3 Sadly, failure to care for our precious commodity can (**a**) place an individual outside of the common "herd" or (**b**) just appear dirty and which may convey a wider social message

The remaining 10–25 % of scalp follicles are small and produce fine **vellus** hairs.

The Terminal Hair Follicle

The terminal hair follicle is not a static organ but undergoes a series of recurrent and prolonged metabolic spurts in which hair is produced. This is followed by a period of involution and a short rest (where usually an old hair is shed) and by another period of prolonged activity when a new hair is grown.

In this section we refer to the anatomy of the follicle during the active growing phase (anagen) and describe later how the anatomy changes as active growth ceases and hairs are shed.

The terminal hair follicle produces a thick and pigmented hair. In the active growing phase (anagen) the follicle consists of a central "command center" deep in the dermis (the papilla) and highly active cells (the matrix) derived from stem cells. The matrix is responsible for creating the hair shaft and the lining of the follicle (the root sheath).

The Papilla

The papilla is comprised of connective tissue and contains a loop of blood vessels to feed the

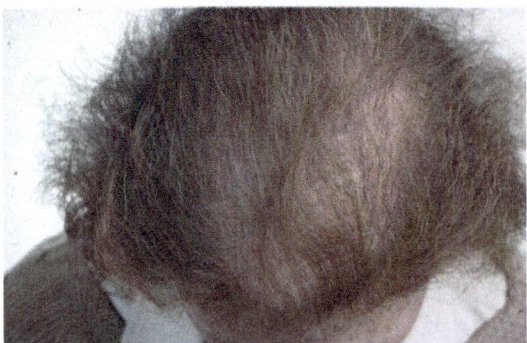

Fig. 1.4 And later—severe diffuse loss across the scalp

matrix cells. Cell division in the papilla is either rare or non-existent but it is responsible for signaling to cells in the dermis for the control of hair growth (Fig. 1.5).

The Matrix
Encasing the papilla, the matrix is a collection of specialized skin epithelial cells often interspersed with the pigment-producing cells, the melanocytes. Active mitosis (cell division) produces the major structures of the hair shaft and the inner root sheath. Almost immediately after they are generated, these cells undergo pre-ordained cell-death (apoptosis) and in so doing express a range of powerful proteins—keratins. These different keratin variants can now be measured and are key markers of hair health (see Chap. 5).

The hair matrix epithelium is one of the fastest growing cell populations in the human body, and is particularly susceptible to chemotherapy or radiotherapy, which kill dividing cells and can result in rapid hair loss (see Chap. 4).

Root Sheath
The root sheath is essentially the lining of the follicle in which the hair grows towards the surface. It is composed of an external and an internal root sheath which is continuous with the outermost layer of the hair fiber. In the upper portion of the follicle a small and probably vestigial muscle inserts into the external sheath—the arrector pili muscle. Above this, the sebaceous gland empties into the space around the hair shaft.

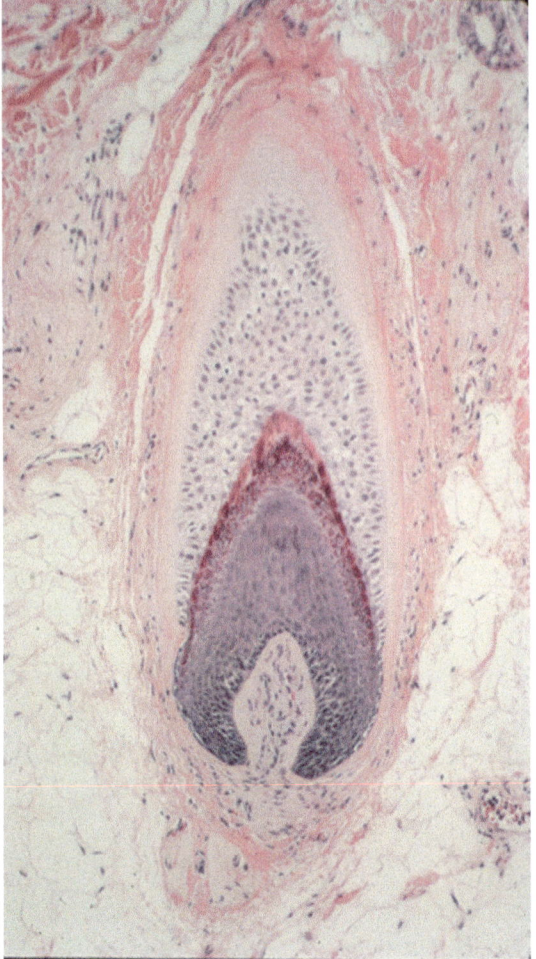

Fig. 1.5 The dermal papilla surrounded by the hair matrix

Stem Cells
Stem cells are undifferentiated multi-potent biological cells that can then differentiate into many different specialized cell lines. Adult stem cells, which are found in various tissues throughout the body, including the hair follicle, maintain the normal turnover of regenerative organs, such as blood, skin, or intestinal tissues.

In the hair follicle, stem cells are found just below the insertion of the arrector pili muscle. Under the influence of the dermal papilla, stem cells migrate downwards into the dermis to create the matrix. Erroneously referred to as the Stem Cell Bulge this area, just below the insertion of the arrector pili muscle is anatomically more

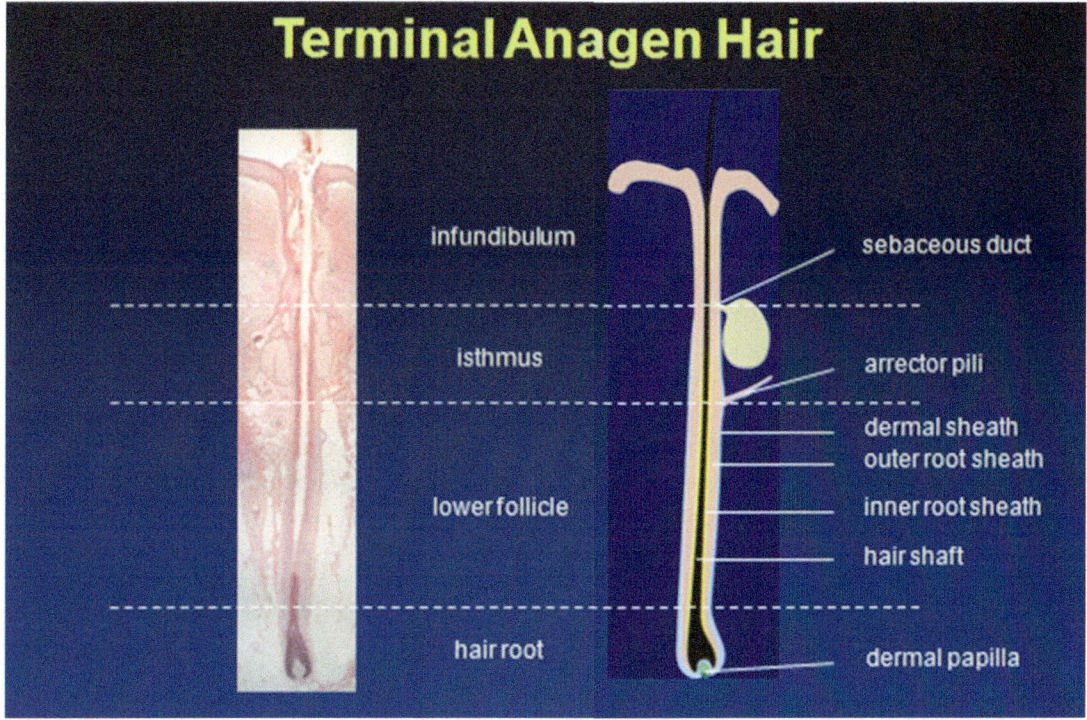

Fig. 1.6 The histology and anatomy of the terminal hair follicle at the height of the growing phase (anagen)

suggestive of a reservoir. Stem cells are also capable of migrating upwards to become skin cells in situations of trauma or burns. Without this reservoir in the hair follicle, the regeneration of the skin after severe burns would be impossible (Fig. 1.6).

The Hair Cycle

As with all mammals, hair does not grow in a continuous manner but in prolonged bursts followed by rests, shedding of the hair shaft and then new growth—the Hair Cycle.

The length of these cycles is determined primarily by individual genetics and by internal and external factors, particularly as we age. Over a lifetime each scalp follicle may grow some 20 separates hairs but with rare exceptions, declining length, diameter, and density.

In the neonatal and early childhood period, hair growth is synchronous. Hairs are shed and start regrowth at the same time. In young children this mass shedding is often observed as a bald patch on the nape of the neck (Fig. 1.7).

Eventually each follicle starts to cycle independently, other than possibly in synchrony with its own immediate group of 2 or 3 follicles. This results in steady and even daily loss across the scalp and prevents mass balding and regrowth.

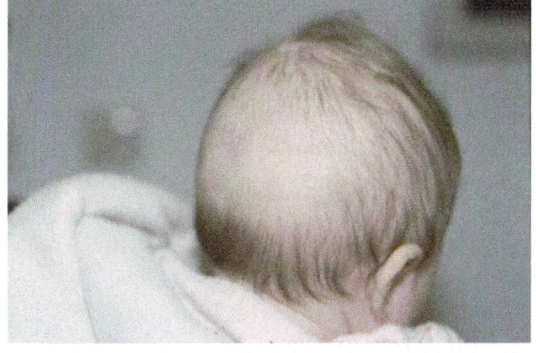

Fig. 1.7 In the neonatal and early childhood period, hair growth is synchronous. As hairs are shed they tend to do so at the same time. In children this mass shedding is often observed as a bald patch on nape of the neck

Anatomical Changes of the Terminal Hair Follicle During Active Growth

The part of the follicle above the arrector pili muscle and the sebaceous gland is permanent and is fixed in the skin. The dermal papilla is also permanent but curiously, is not fixed anatomically. The area between the insertion of the arrector pili muscle and the dermal papilla is not structurally permanent but is formed as the follicle moves from a resting to a growing phase. Current theory proposes that when the follicle cell enters a period of active growth (anagen) a subset of the stem population moves down to associate with the dermal papilla and forms the matrix from which both the hair shaft and the lining of the follicle—the inner and outer root sheaths—are produced. At this stage the hair bulb composed of the dermal papilla and matrix is approximately 4–5 mm deep in the dermis. The fully formed hair bulb is highly imbued with blood vessels, nerves, and lymphatics.

The dermal papilla controls the initiation of anagen by communication with cells in the dermis. The hormone prostaglandin is involved in the communication but the exact mechanism is still not fully understood. The matrix becomes self-sustaining throughout this part of the cycle. It is probable that the pigment producing cells—the melanocytes—move like the follicle stem cells and only repopulate he matrix during anagen. They are highly important cells in the whole cycle and are crucial for a healthy hair follicle.

Phases of the Hair Cycle: Anagen/Catagen/Telogen/Exogen

The length of anagen is determined by the individual's genetics and for most of the population is within in the 2–6 year range. When active growth ceases (for reasons unknown) there is a short pause (catagen) where after the follicle involutes and produces a resting hair with a bead visible to the naked eye, There is a pause in the cycle of some 3 months and the follicle is termed to be in a telogen phase. This telogen hair is eventually shed and the characteristic bead like structure can be seen with the naked eye particularly on dark clothing. This bead (Fig. 1.9b) is often, but erroneously, thought to be the hair root. By comparison the plucked hair root is elongated and "juicy" (see Fig. 1.9a).

Until recently it was thought that the resting hair was removed by grooming or was physically pushed out the follicle by a new hair growing behind it. Recent research suggests that there may also be a specific shedding mechanism (exogen) and often the follicle is occupied by both a resting and a growing hair (Fig. 1.8).

When the actively growing hair is removed by pulling (depilation) the dermal papilla remains in the follicle to generate a new hair and a long anagen root is seen. It is from this anagen hair root that DNA can be extracted (Figs. 1.9 and 1.10).

Interruption of Hair Growth

Hair growth may be interrupted during the growing phase resulting in a sudden or gradual excess loss of hairs (effluvium). A shift in the proportion of hairs growing to resting (anagen to telogen) results in an increase in shed telogen hairs (telogen effluvium) tantamount to a moult. Common causes include severe and sudden weight loss, severe illness or post operatively. A natural telogen effluvium often occurs after childbirth due to the abrupt cessation of anagen in hairs which under the influence of oestrogens, are in synchronised anagen.

See Chap. 4 for further causes of hair loss.

Kenogen

There is a lag time (kenogen) between the cessation of the manufacture of one hair and the recommencement of growth of a new one. This lag time increases with age which adds to naturally diminishing volume over time.

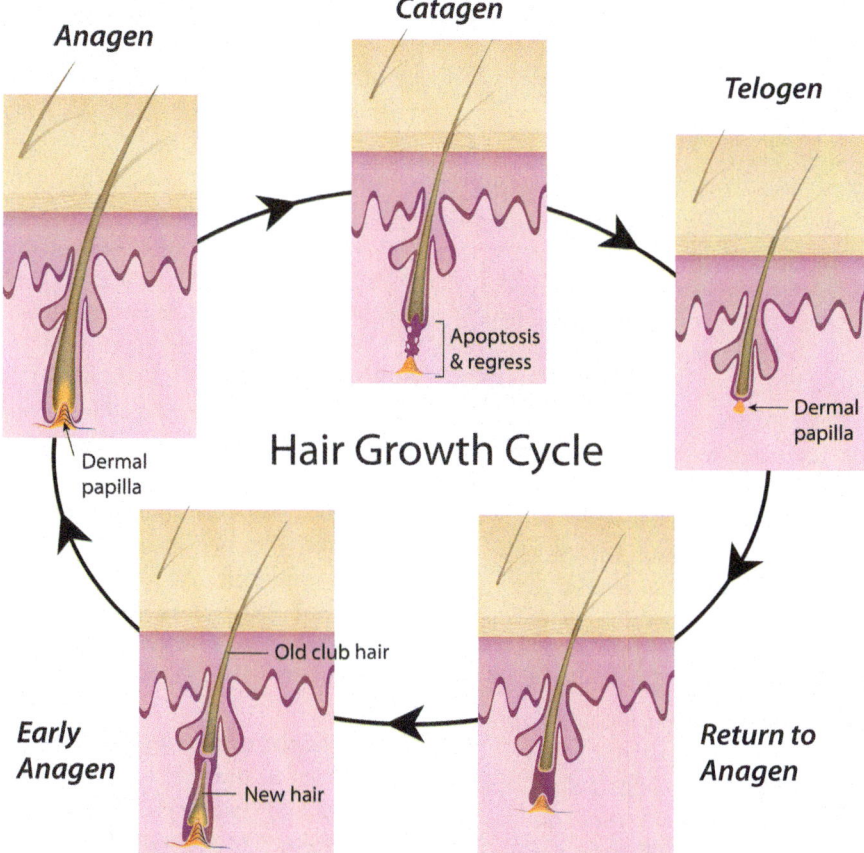

Fig. 1.8 Graphic of the hair cycle—exogen not included

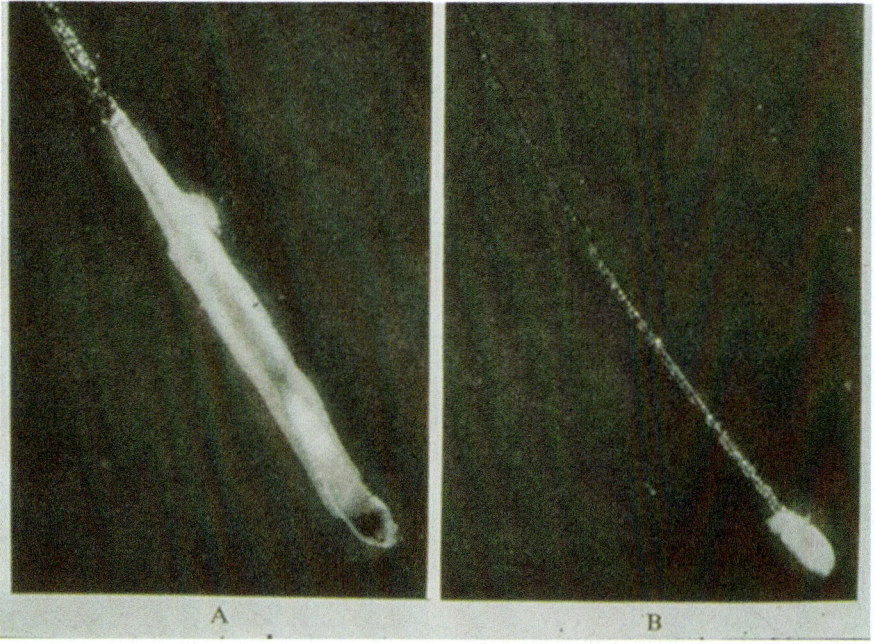

Fig. 1.9 (**a**) A plucked hair reveals the anagen root (*left*) compared to (**b**) a hair which has been naturally shed showing the telogen bulb. The plucked hair contains all human DNA and is critical for forensic investigation. The telogen hair does not contain DNA

Science Box
Growth Rate Facts
- Anagen varies between 2 and 6 years but tends to shorten with age. Depending on genetics – may be up to 10 years
- In infants the hair cycle is synchronized but in the first year of life, this is partially lost until in adulthood follicles are capable of cycling independent of the adjoining follicles.
- Under normal circumstances approximately 90–95 % of scalp hairs are in anagen and 5–10 % in telogen.
- Each human scalp hair grows at 0.9 cm per month or approximately 11 cm per year.
- Total daily hair production is in the order of 5 m per day.
- The result of continuous growth from (say) 100,000 follicles is the production of over 11 km of hair per year.
- An anagen phase of 6 years results in a head of hair equivalent to a 66 km. Natural hair loss is 50–80 hairs per day, mostly when washing or grooming. The longer and darker the hair, the more apparent loss is observed.

Most of the other areas of the body grow virtually colorless and thin (less than 40 µm) hairs—vellus hairs.

After puberty, both sexes may grow terminal hairs in areas associated with sexual signaling and activity plus variable body hair. There are significant regional differences with significantly less body hair in East Asian peoples.

Follicle Density

Scalp follicles are arranged in groups of two, three, four, and vary rarely five (follicular units) with three the commonest (Fig. 1.11).

It has been postulated that in fetal skin, there may be one primary unit and others develop around it. At birth the total life time number of follicles is already present and as the skin stretches with growth, density inevitably decreases.

The Concept of the Aging of Hair

The tissues of the scalp and hair follicle inevitably age and their activity decline. The proliferative tissues in the hair matrix are subject to the intrinsic factors associated with constant metabolic activity and natural (chronological) aging. In addition external (extrinsic) factors may also impact on the quality of hair produced. These factors inevitably occur in conjunction and are cumulative over time.

Intrinsic factors are overwhelmingly inherited and result in, for instance, male pattern balding and premature graying. Extrinsic factors include the effects of ultraviolet radiation (UVR), smoking, and possibly, nutrition.

As a result of continuous metabolic activity, highly reactive oxygen molecules (ROS) are generated in the cells leading to oxidative stress which is now believed to play a major role in the aging process. The damaging effects of these ROS are both induced from the mitochondria in the matrix cells and melanocytes and externally from the environment. The follicle possesses enzymes and vitamins (E and C) which help to quench the ROS. Eventually, the ROS overwhelm the defenses leading to damage to the active cells. The effects of this are seen as graying, and an imperceptible but steady decrease in hair production both in terms of quantity and quality.

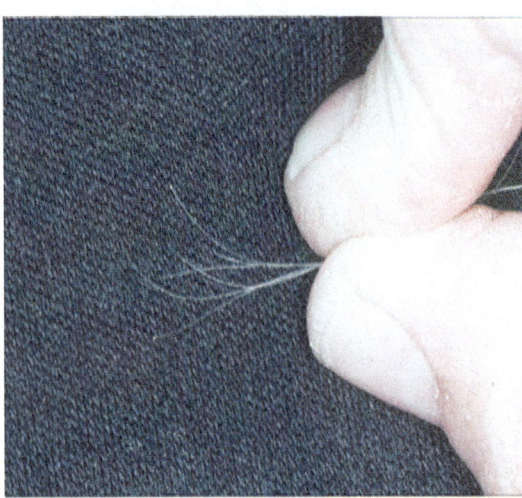

Fig. 1.10 Telogen hairs showing the characteristic bulbs—invariably mistaken for the root. We naturally lose between 50 and 80 such hairs each day usually when shampooing and brushing

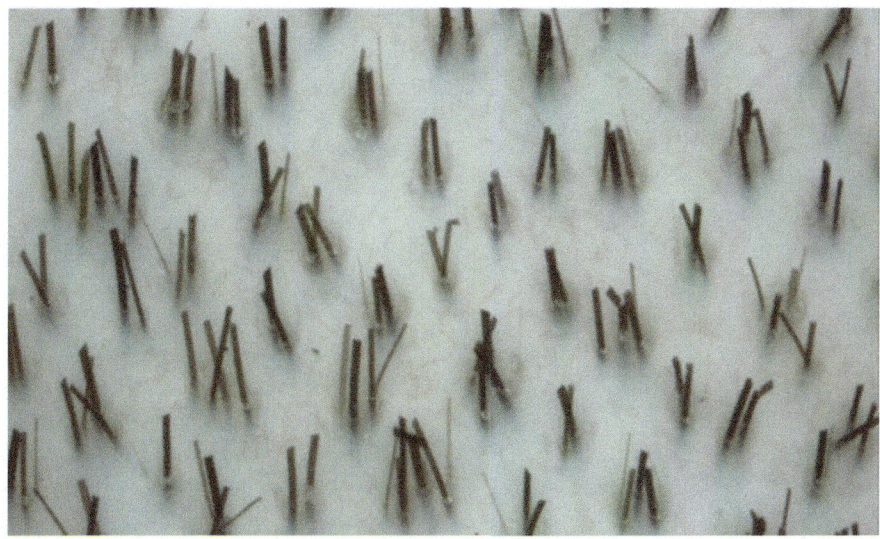

Fig. 1.11 Follicular grouping on the scalp

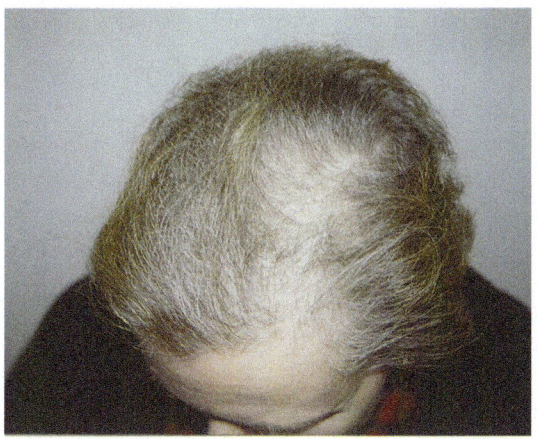

Fig. 1.12 Tangible loss of bulk and visible scalp—signs of hair thinning

Hair Thinning: Reducing Hair Density, Diameter, and Hair Mass

A common complaint of women as they age is that of losing hair density or in common parlance—thinning.

This may be manifest as a tangible loss of bulk, visible scalp, or reduction in the volume of a pony tail (Fig. 1.12).

It is often difficult for an observer, stylist, or dermatologist to interpret early thinning, particularly if there is no evidence of greater than normal daily hair loss. Sadly, by the time this reduction in total hair mass is apparent, some 50 % loss of hairs may have occurred (Fig. 1.13).

Hair Density

At all ages, there is a wide and normally distributed scatter of hairs over the scalp.

Possibly as a result of the impact of ROS described above, density in women gradually declines from 293 cm^{-2} plus/minus at 35 to 211 cm^{-2} plus/minus at age 70.

Hair Diameter

Mean hair diameter increases from age 22 to a peak in the mid-thirties but gradually declines with advancing age. In addition some follicles cease functioning altogether (Fig. 1.14).

Allied to this concept is that of hair shaft "aging." Hair as it emerges from the follicular opening is in its most perfect state. As this growth progresses, the hair shaft quality deteriorates "ages" due to external factors such as environmental, chemical, and physical insults. The process is known as weathering (see Chap. 3) and is the most common hair disorder encountered by women.

The combined effect of the intrinsic and extrinsic factors at a follicular level and extrinsic aging of the shaft is to render the hair thinner, weaker, and less "healthy."

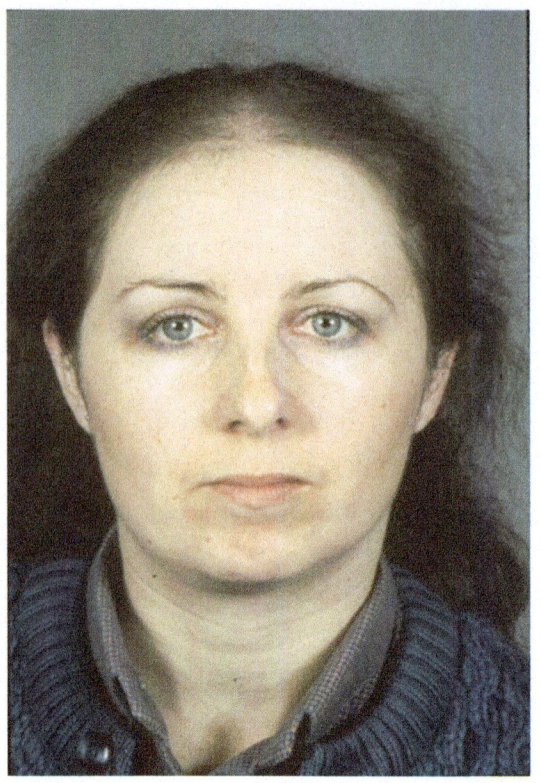

Fig. 1.13 Visible scalp indicates up to 50 % hair loss

As an individual ages, the keratin production slows and the hair shaft becomes thinner with a mean diameter of terminal hairs. Finally, the interval between cessation of growth of one hair and the commencement of a new (kenogen) extends.

All these factors contribute to a gradual reduction in hair mass caused by reduced numbers of hairs, reduced diameters, and extended intervals of growth. It explains the common complaint of "I had such a head of hair when I was young – look at it now." This perception or reality of reduced hair density can have a major impact on the self-perception of healthy hair and self-esteem.

Research carried out at the University of Sheffield by Professor Andrew Messenger and Dr Pattie Burke [1] demonstrated that high diameter hairs but at low density are not perceived as hair loss. Alternatively, smaller diameter hairs with normal density tend to be interpreted as reduced density (Fig. 1.15).

Hair Growth and Nutrition

Hair growth requires amino acids to form the protein keratin. A normal "balanced" diet is

Age (Indo-European Women)	Average Hair Density (hairs/cm2)	Delta (%) in density Vs age 30
30	290	
40	270	-6.8
50	263	-9.3
60	235	-18.9
70	211	-27.2
80	185	-36.2

Fig. 1.14 Mean hair diameter increases from age 22 to a peak in the mid-thirties but gradually declines with advancing age

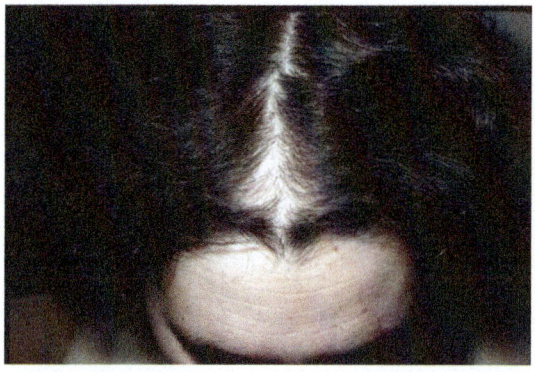

Fig. 1.15 Female pattern hair loss—the classic presentation—showing the "Christmas tree" effect

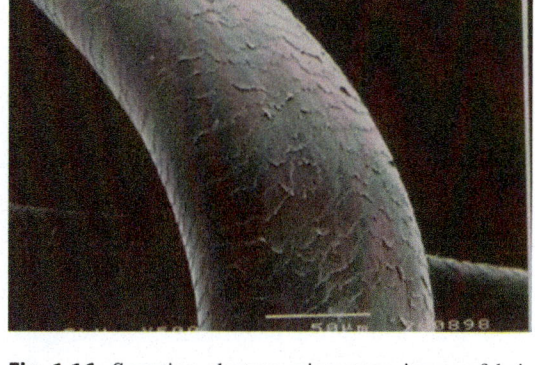

Fig. 1.16 Scanning electron microscope image of hair shaft

more than adequate to sustain normal hair growth. Even in times reduced food intake (as in sensible dieting) there is no scientific evidence that there is any interruption with normal hair production.

Again there is no strong scientific evidence that the plethora of oral hair supplements including vitamins and ferritin have any effect on improving hair production in healthy individuals. Further, there is no strong evidence that they have any clinical effect in hair loss states.

Crash dieting with rapid reduction in the Body Mass Index is associated with reports of hair loss due to telogen effluvium (see Chap. 4).

Hair: The Cosmetic Aspects

The result of this hair growth activity is the production of a terminal hair shaft. This may be described, like the carapace of a crustacean, as a filamentous biomaterial since it contains no living matter or possesses any bio-feedback mechanisms. There is no pain if it is cut nor does cutting it make it grow stronger or thicker. From this point on, whatever happens to the hair shaft, is regarded as cosmetic "which includes beauty, esthetics, or appearance." In reality, modern research has identified that behind these cosmetic changes, there are structural and measurable changes to the very core of the hair (see Chap. 3).

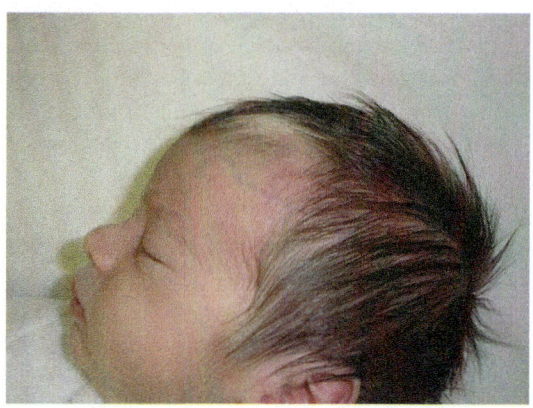

Fig. 1.17 Lanugo hair seen on the face of this newborn

The Terminal Hair Shaft

A single human hair is merely a bundle of compressed protein with a small quantity of fats and traces of minerals and vitamins. It contains no living cells and receives no support other than mechanical from the follicle. The visible hair shaft has no active metabolism yet in combination with its neighbors can exude an almost mystical vitality and strength. Weight for weight hair is stronger than steel (Fig. 1.16).

There are three essential types of hair in humans which are age related and dependant to some extent on the size of the follicle.

Lanugo hair—is fine and non-medullated hair which appears on the fetus and with rare exceptions is shed prior or immediately after birth (Fig. 1.17).

Vellus hair is fine, short, and non- or lightly pigmented hair (less than 40 μm in diameter) and is the most numerous of human hairs. It can be seen from the neonatal period onwards covering all surfaces other than the palms and soles of the feet. At puberty, some vellus hairs enlarge to become terminal hairs and develop sebaceous glands. Vellus hairs occur on the scalp but are far less numerous than terminal hairs (see below).

In male and female pattern hair loss, terminal hairs miniaturize and return to the size of vellus hairs. This can be reversed with treatment (see Chap. 4).

Terminal hair—thick, long, and pigmented. The terminal hair is some 50–150 μm thick. Terminal hairs are the dominant hairs on the scalp, eyebrows, lashes, axillae, and genital areas. In men terminal hairs are variably found on the trunk and legs. There is great regional difference in terminal body hairs. It is relatively uncommon in Oriental areas and more common in Indo-Europeans.

The cross section of the hair terminal shaft reveals three major components:

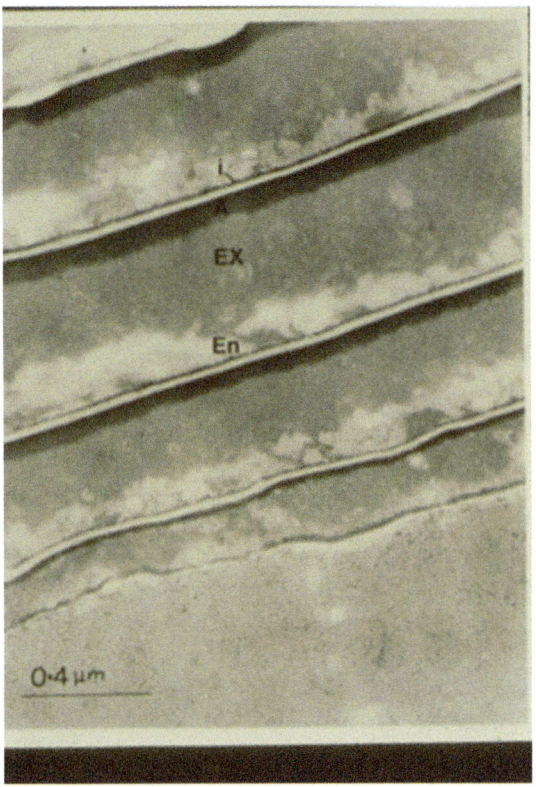

Fig. 1.18 Overlapping scales of the cuticle

- the cuticle—the outer protective layer
- the cortex—the massive core of the hair
- the medulla—a central soft protein core which is more common in thicker hair and particularly so in white hairs

The main constituents of these structures are sulfur-rich proteins, lipids, water, melanin, and trace elements.

The Cuticle

The cuticle is composed of specialized keratins and consists of six to eight layers of flattened overlapping cells with their free edges directed upward to the tip of the hair shaft. There are several layers to each cell—the innermost endocuticle is covered by the exocuticle which lies closer to the external surface and is comprised of three parts: the b-layer, the a-layer, and the epicuticle. The b-layer and the a-layer are largely protein. The epicuticle is a hydrophobic (water resistant) lipid layer of 18-methyleicosanoic acid attached by a covalent chemical bond to the surface of the fiber. This is commonly known as the f-layer.

The f-layer is of critical importance to hair health and its fate is discussed in following chapters.

The cuticle's complex structure allows it to slide as the hair swells and the f-layer imbues a considerable degree of water resistance (hydrophobicity). It is critical in protecting the hair and rendering it resistant to the influx and outflow of moisture (Fig. 1.18).

The normal cuticle has a smooth appearance, allowing light reflection and limiting friction between the hair shafts. It is primarily responsible for the luster and texture of the hair (Fig. 1.19).

Hair: The Cosmetic Aspects

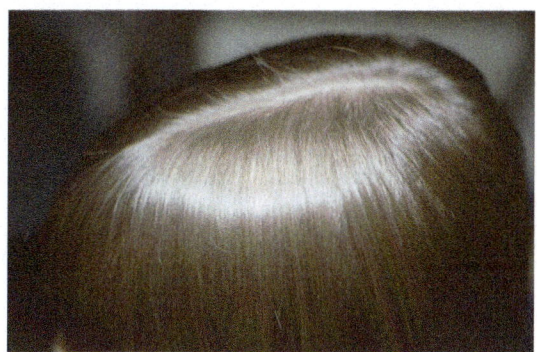

Fig. 1.19 Healthy hair—reflection from the intact cuticles of well aligned hair is largely responsible for hair shine

The cuticle may be damaged by four different "insult" sources. Environmental, mechanical, chemical, and heat (see Chap. 3).

Chemical removal of the f-layer particularly by oxidation during bleaching or perming eliminates the first hydrophobic defence and leaves the hair more porous and vulnerable. If the cuticle is damaged there is little change in the tensile properties of hair; however, its protective function is diminished (see Chap. 3) (Fig. 1.20).

The Cortex

The cortex forms the main bulk of a fully formed (keratinized) hair shaft and contributes almost all the mechanical properties of the hair, particularly strength and elasticity.

The cortex consists of closely pack spindle shaped cells rich in keratin filaments comprising 400–500 amino acid residues paired together to form proto-filaments which make up a keratin chain. These are orientated parallel to the long axis of the hair shaft and embedded in an amorphous matrix of high sulfur proteins. The keratin chains have a large number of sulfur-containing cystine bonds which create a strong cross link between adjacent chains. These so-called disulfide bonds are critical in conferring confer shape, stability, and resilience to the hair shaft, and can only be broken by external oxidative chemical

The f- Layer

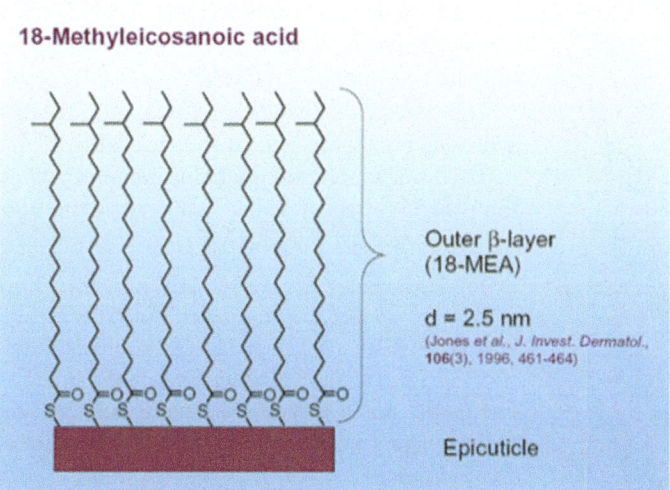

- Covalently bound, mono-molecular layer of a unique, branched, fatty acid – 18 methyl eicosanoic acid (18mea).
- 18mea, combined with the underlying protein (epicuticle) of hair keratin is termed the f-layer.

Fig. 1.20 Preservation of the outer f-layer is of critical importance in maintaining "hair health" or homeostasis. Removal renders the hair shaft potentially vulnerable to further damage

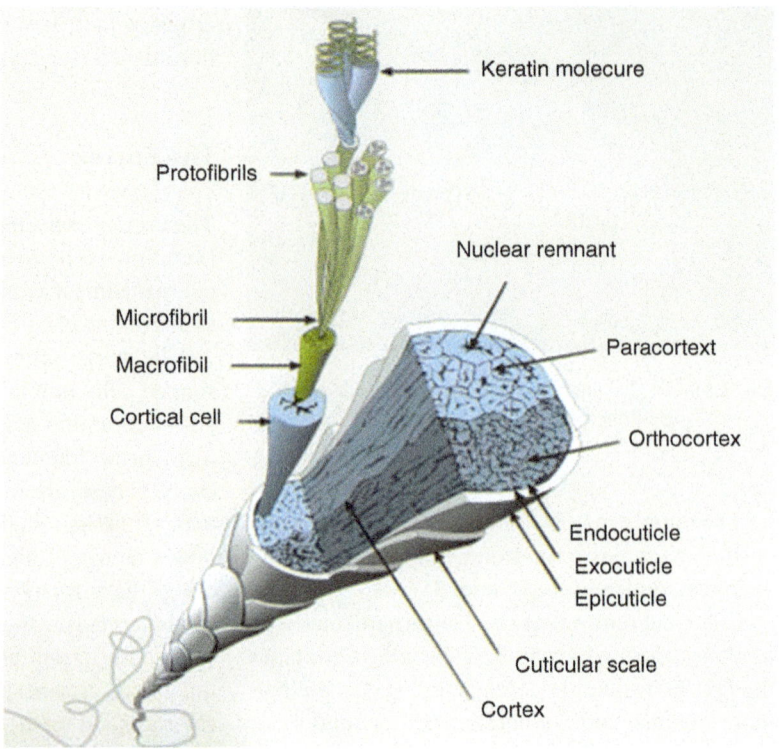

Fig. 1.21 Graphic to demonstrate the composition of the cortex

agents such as occurs with perming or relaxing (Fig. 1.21).

Weak hydrogen bonds and salt links link the keratin polypeptide chains together. These weaker bonds are easily overcome by water rendering curly hair, temporarily, straight.

The powerful disulfide bonds and weaker hydrogen bonds are crucial to hair health.

The cortex contains melanin granules which color the fiber based on the number, distribution, and types of melanin granules (Fig. 1.22).

The Medulla

The medulla is a soft proteinaceous core present in thicker and white hair. It has no known function in humans.

Abnormal Hairs

Sadly, not all hairs are "normal." Genetically inherited hair diseases may produce abnormal hairs which result in weakness and/or major

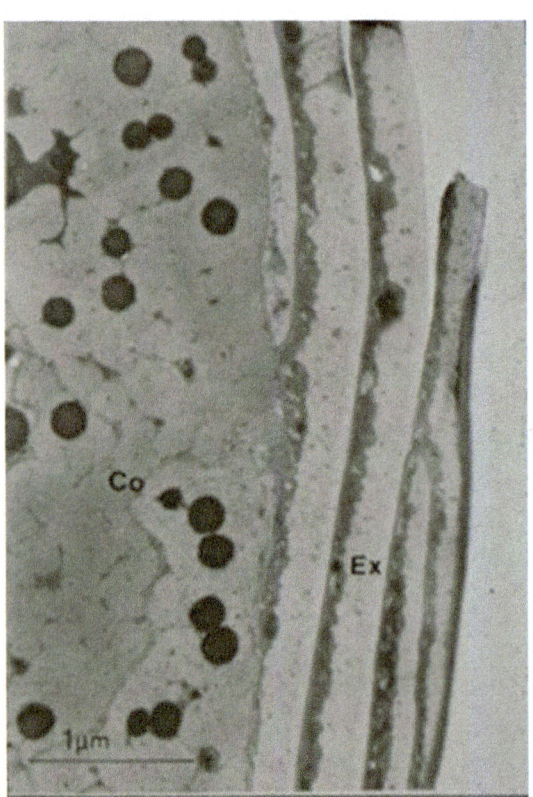

Fig. 1.22 Melanin granules in the cortex with overlapping scales of the cuticle

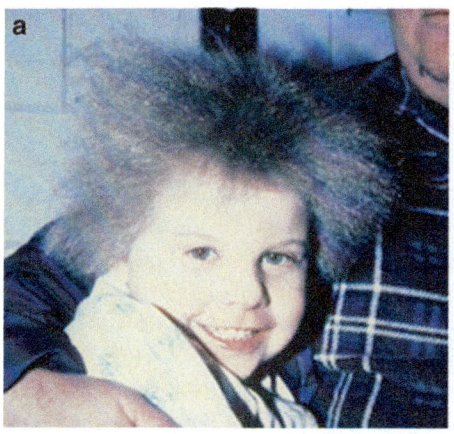 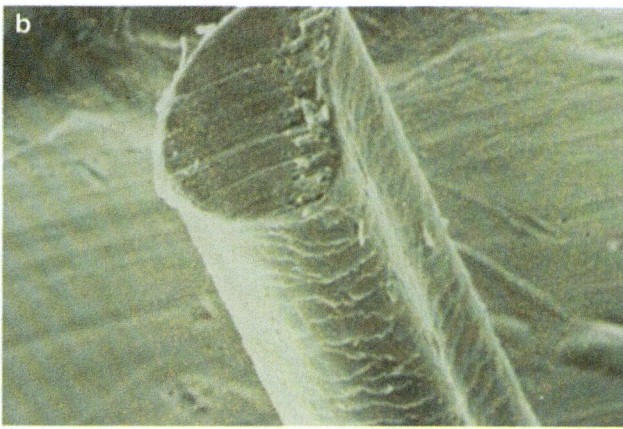

Fig. 1.23 (**a**) Uncombable hair due to (**b**) abnormality of the hair shafts

problems in grooming. One such example is cheveaux incoiffable (uncombable hair syndrome)—see below (Fig. 1.23).

Hair Diameter and Texture

The diameter of human hair varies from 17 to 180 μm (0.00067 to 0.0071 in.). Hair less than 40 μm is regarded as vellus hair.

Hair texture is a less precise term but is usually classified as follows:

Fine	Less than 60 μm
Medium	60–80 μm
Thick	80–150 μm

Many women on questioning, believe their hair to be finer than accurate measuring would confirm. This misunderstanding may affect their less than ideal, choice of hair care products.

Hair Types

Not all terminal hairs are the same shape (phenotype).

Terminal hairs have traditionally been described as round, oval, or flat. In reality there is a broad spectrum of hair shapes and although individuals tend to bear essentially one type on their scalps it has been observed that all three can be present. The phenotype is determined by genetic inheritance and different forms on one head has become more common with increasing genetic diversity due to the breakdown of social and ethnic barriers in societies.

Whilst peoples from sub-equatorial Africa and their dispersed descendants have hair follicles which are curved, the final shape of the hair emerging from the follicle is more determined by the activity of the matrix cells deep in the follicle and the manner in which the keratin proteins are laid down in the cortex.

The hypothesis that hair shaft shape is principally due to the shape of the follicle is further confounded by the ability of terminal hair follicles to produce different phenotypes under altered circumstances. Patients after chemotherapy routinely report dramatic change in hair shaft phenotypes, presumably due to a change in arrangements of keratins in the cortex from a "reprogrammed" matrix.

Phenotype and "Hair Health"

The shape of the shaft(s) has significant implications for long-term hair health. Increased susceptibility of the cuticle to physical damage is more common in flatter hair. The greater the diameter of the cortex, the greater the resistance of the hair shaft to environmental and self-inflicted damage (see Chap. 3). These considerations are of fundamental importance when designing hair care products and regimens.

Classification of Hair Phenotypes

Classically, hair shaft shape (phenotype) was described as caucasoid, negroid, or mongaloid, supposedly alluding to inhabitants or descendants of people from Europe, Africa, or "Asia."

This classification presupposed that these groups of related peoples were regionally static or evolved in parallel isolation. In reality, from a genetic standpoint peoples living north of the equator have considerable affinity with "European" and Middle East genotypes and phenotypes. Asia is even more problematic and is further complicated by linguistic and commercial imperatives. The majority of peoples from the north of the Indian subcontinent, they have a much greater genetic and phenotypic association with Europeans than with the relatively static populations in East Asia.

Science Note

In the medical sciences, there is great debate as to whether racial categorizations as broad as Caucasian are valid. Several journals (e.g., *Nature Genetics*, *Archives of Pediatrics & Adolescent Medicine*, and the *British Medical Journal*) have issued guidelines stating that researchers should carefully define their populations, and avoid broad-based social constructions—because these categories would more likely measure differences in socioeconomic class and access to medical treatment that disproportionately affect minority groups, rather than "racial" differences. The term race in itself when applied to homo sapiens, is genetically irrelevant.

This author contends that this classification is now archaic and was based on a number of racial notions, stereotypes, and prejudices which are no longer acceptable nor have any genetic basis.

A more phenotypic subgroup approach might be proposed as below whilst recognising that there is still room for linguistic difficulties. The proposal is based on traditional usage in English.

Sub-equatorial African—a unique phenotype with the hair shaft flattened and prone to tight curling. It is evident that despite considerable genetic diversity for peoples living south of the Equator in Africa, this phenotype is imperative and probably a response to the environment. Displaced descendants of these peoples have carried this phenotype into the wider world. In the USA although many people have this phenotype, there is considerable gene mixing. Many Australasian – indigenous people of Australia

East Asian—circular and of wide diameter with a tendency to straightness and rigidity.

Indo-European/Continental European—more ovoid and of variable characteristics—thin/straight to thicker and/or wavy/curly. A more practical approach derived from recent research is a simple descriptor. Thin, thick, straight, curly or colored hair and irrespective of genotype or region.

Sub-Equatorial African Hair

The hair shaft is typically flattened and prone to curl. It is particularly vulnerable to physical damage and tends to require particular attention to moisturizing.

The distribution of African hair is strongly orientated towards the equator and is the most dominant expression of this hair phenotype. Research indicates that although sub-Saharan Africans are the most genetically diverse group on Earth, Afro-textured hair is the overwhelming hair type. This suggests a strong, selective pressure and does not seem to support sexual selection as the sole or principal cause of this distribution.

Sub-equatorial hair was exported to both the Americas in the 1800s and into Europe from post colonial Africa in the twentieth century. Of all the hair types it suffers most from grooming issues due to its dense curl and from breakage due to its shape. In addition, washing frequency is much lower than with other hair types due to its unique nature and combined with water resource issues (Fig. 1.24).

Many African women now relax their hair for both practical and esthetic reasons. This in turn brings issues of damage. African hair has required as we shall see in later chapters, a paradigm shift in product development.

Fig. 1.24 Durban South Africa—(**a**) classical sub-equatorial African hair plus hair dye and (**b**) braids, relaxing, extensions and a "No. 1" haircut—strategies for coping

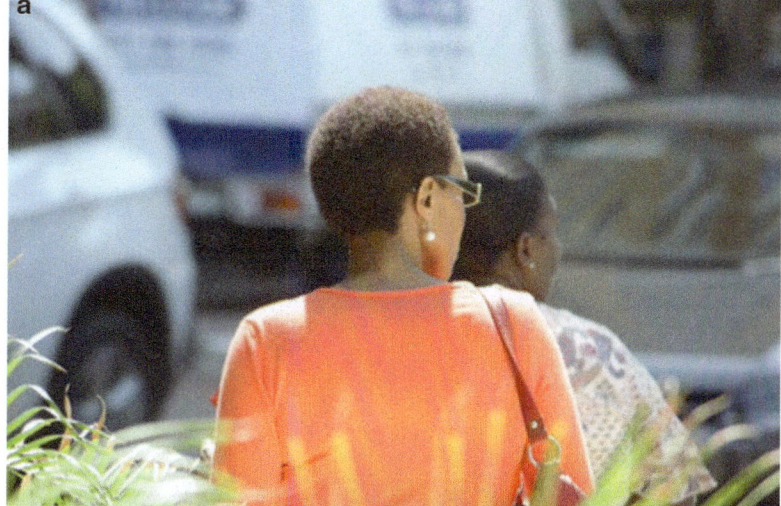

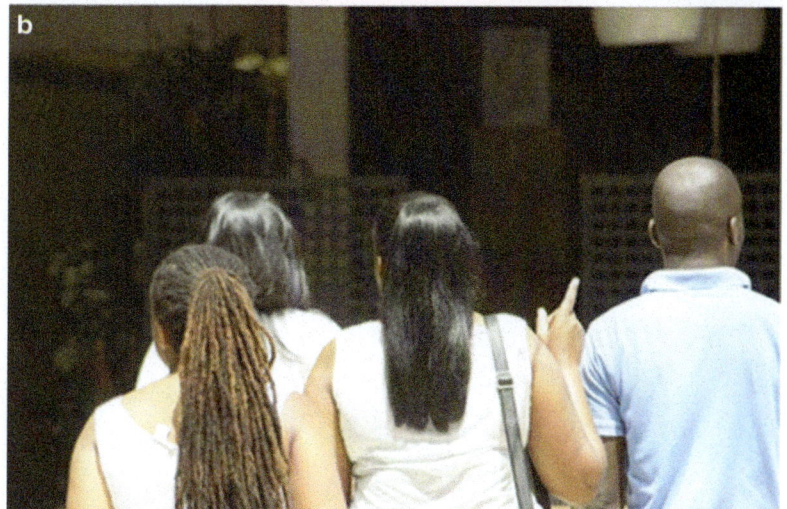

Australasian Hair

Genetic evidence shows the Aborigineal peoples' ancestors arrived in Australia, some 50,000 years ago and remained isolated until Captain Cook discovered their land.

They are direct descendants of the first modern humans to leave Africa, without any genetic mixture from other subgroups. Their highly pigmented skin reflects an African origin and a migration and residence in latitudes near the equator, unlike Europeans and Asians whose ancestors gained the paler skin necessary for living in northern latitudes.

Based on the rate of mutation in DNA, geneticists estimate that the Aborigineal peoples split from the ancestors of all Eurasians some 70,000 years ago, and that the ancestors of Europeans and East Asians split from each other about 30,000 years ago.

Their hair is interesting in having features of sub-equatorial Africa but with a distinct loosening of the tight curl. Interestingly, some Aborigine children are born with blonde hair (Fig. 1.25).

East Asian Straight Hair

Classical hair in East/SW Asia is thick (up to 150 μm), essentially straight, and black. A quarter

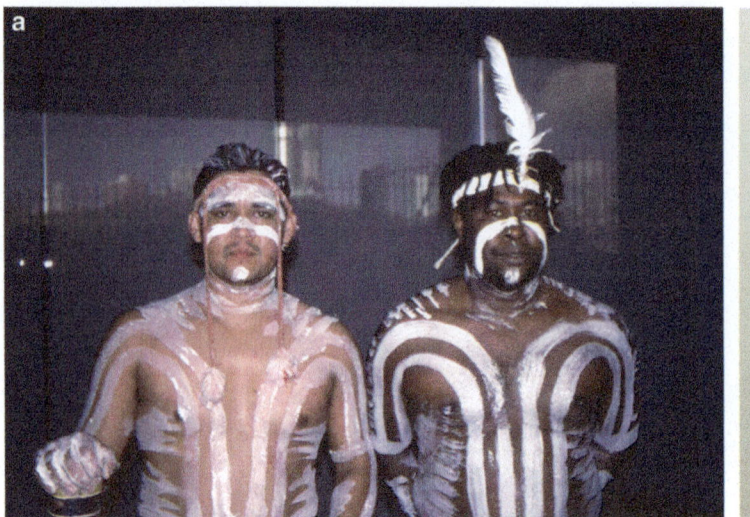 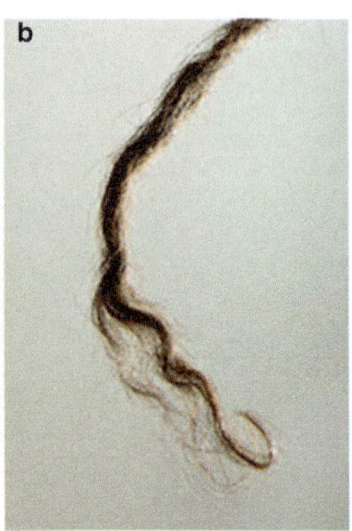

Fig. 1.25 (**a**) Australasian hair is interesting in having features of sub-equatorial Africa but (**b**) with a distinct loosening of the tight curl

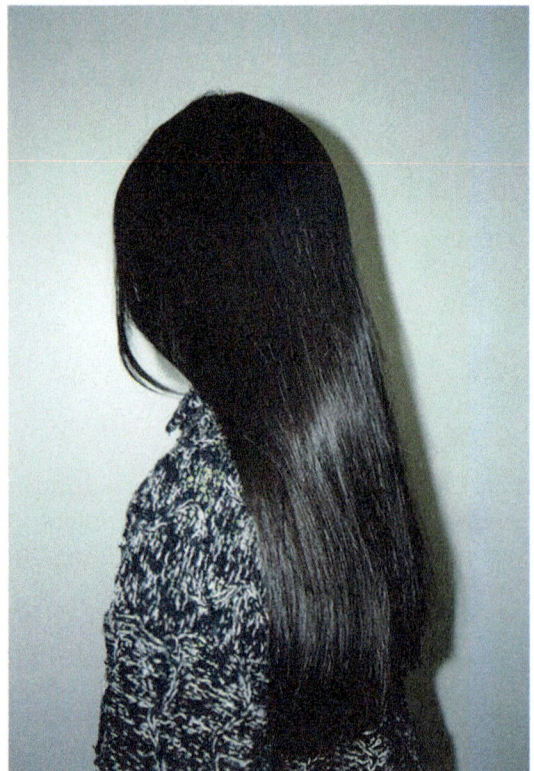

Fig. 1.26 Straight black hair is the commonest expression of homo sapiens hair thick, straight, and darkly pigmented with eumelanin. Control of excess volume may be an issue

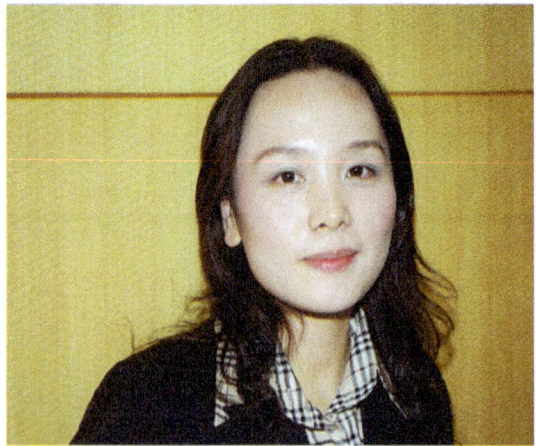

Fig. 1.27 Not all eastern and south eastern asian peoples have straight hair or the thick hair associated with the extreme north east and Inuit peoples

of the world's population carry this phenotype descendant groups (Fig. 1.26).

However, not all such peoples have straight or thick hair associated with the extreme north east and Inuit peoples. The range of hair diameters stretches from 80 to 150 with a South to North bias of increasing diameter (Fig. 1.27).

Volume control is an issue, and perming is still widely utilized as a method of control. Shine is a key requirement but widespread bleaching of highly pigmented hair brings significant damage issues to those who wish to follow celebrity "trends."

Indo-European/Continental European Hair

The broad group of Indo-Europeans shows an East to West bias of darkly pigmented, straight hair to thinner, lighter hair. The Indian subcontinent has hair classically straight. In Europe a range of straight, wavy, and curly hair occurs. The presence of lighter shades and blondes associated with pheomelanin pigment increases in the NW of Europe (Fig. 1.28).

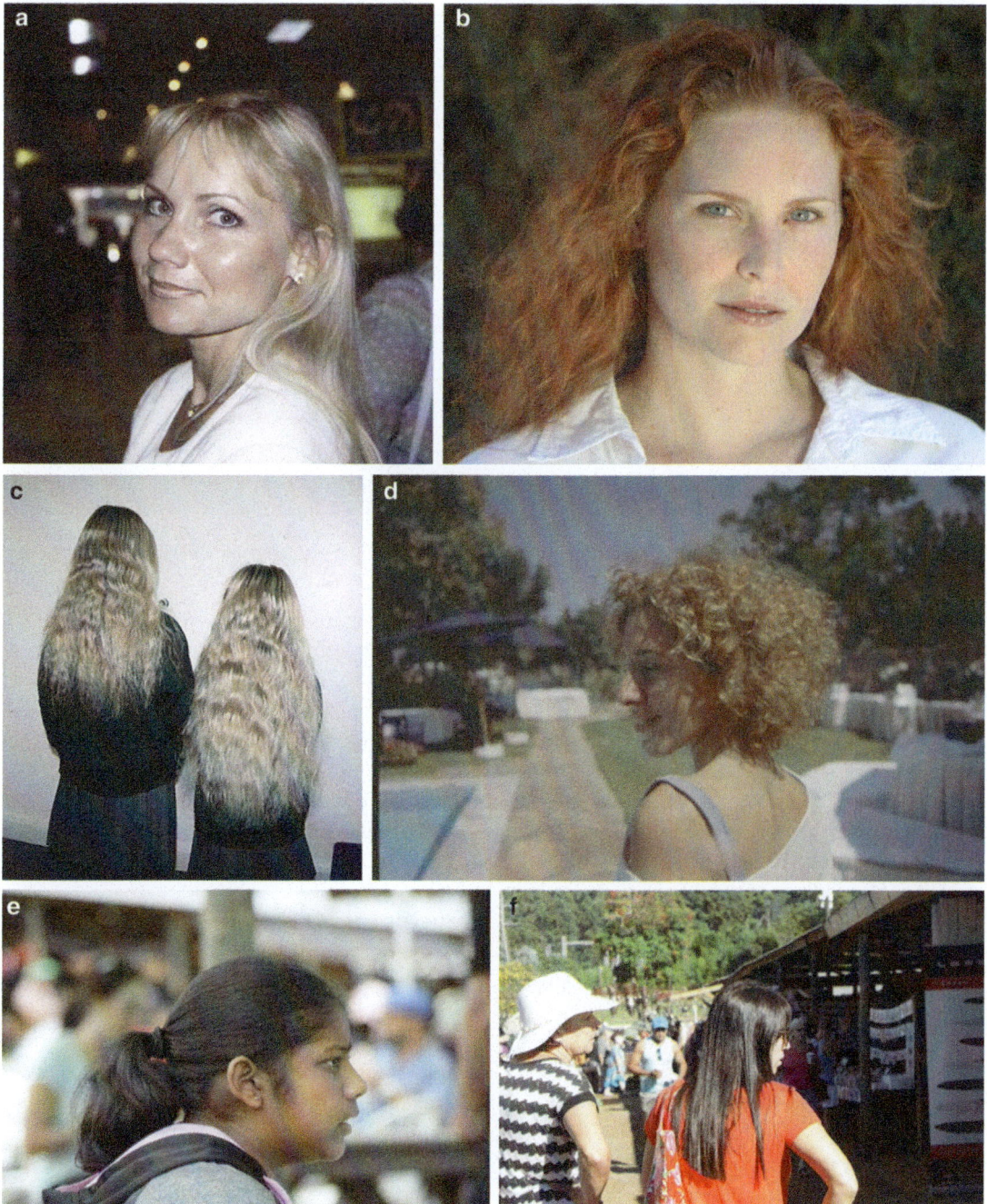

Fig. 1.28 Hair types within the Indo-European/Continental European range—(**a**) Nordic fine blonde; (**b**) the red of pheomelanin; (**c**) twins with identical wave patterns; (**d**) tight curls from Greece; (**e**) Indian girl in South Africa; (**f**) Indian girl with probable "keratin "treatment

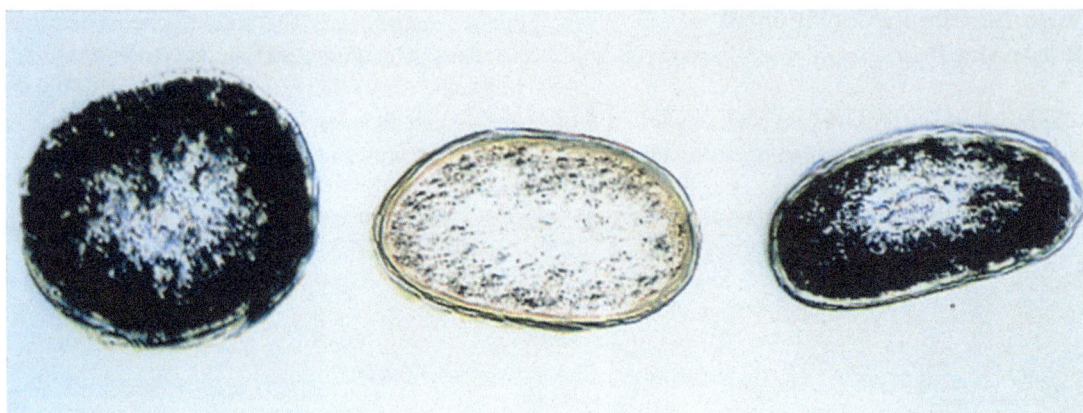

Fig. 1.29 East Asian/Indo-European, and African hair shaft phenotypes—the round darkly pigmented hair of the orient, the more oval hair of Indo-Europeans and the flattened hair of sub-Saharan Africa

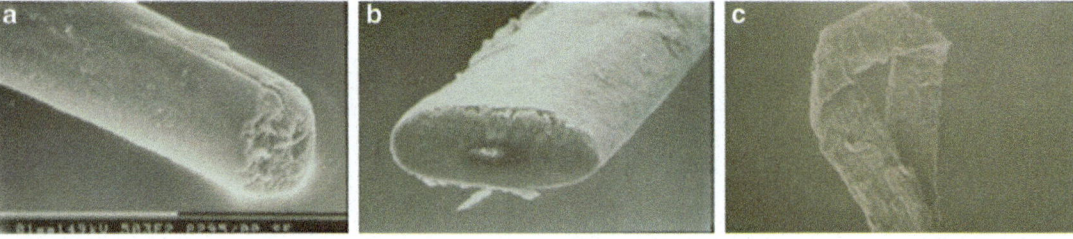

Fig. 1.30 (**a–c**) EMGS—the "classical" three different hair phenotypes—illustrating not only the diameter differences but the tendency of African hair to curl

As human beings spread out around the world, arrival in Europe only occurred in the last 35,000 years. Low sunlight levels are regarded as the cause of the emergence of lightened skins but why light hair is uncertain. Only 1.8 % of humans have naturally light/blond hair with the highest preponderance in Estonia.

Indo-European hair diameter tends to be in the lower to middle range and Eastern Asian hair in the upper. The combination of hair diameter and shape contributes significantly to the general behavior of hair and consequently its cosmetic management.

Hair Phenotypes in the Americas

It is accepted that this proposed nomenclature is far from all embracing and is particularly problematic for the Americas. The indigenous peoples of both North and South America were descendants of Inuits who entered Alaska across the Bering Straits some 12,000 years ago and presumably had hair characteristics of East Asian peoples. Waves of immigration of peoples from particularly Europe and Africa have produced increasing complexity and latterly wider gene sharing (Figs. 1.29 and 1.30).

Developments of Human Hair Differences

Despite the apparent phenotypic differences, all modern humans are of a single race derived from a single female ancestor (African Eve) and a single male ancestor (African Adam) although they did not live at the same time.

The exact hair shape (phenotype) of our early hominid predecessors is unknown. It is presumed that during the gradual process by which our immediate ancestor Homo erectus began a transition from furry to "naked" skin, hair texture changed from straight hair (the condition of most mammals, including all apes). The potential for a more wavy form or even curled phenotype arrived with modern humans and is assumed to be the result of environmental pressures and/or sexual selection.

It is not certain at what point classical sub-equatorial African tightly curled hair evolved

> **Science Box**
>
> The curly hair phenotype is universal in sub-equatorial peoples but only 15 % of Indo-Europeans express curls.

but it may be a late development due to climatic changes.

Straight hair appears to be a new trait in human evolution and is associated with newly emerged genetic alternatives (alleles) in both the genes which provide strength to the hair follicle—trichohyalin (TCHH) and a gene which is important for synthesizing proteins the EDAR gene. This latter gene is common in East Asians but not in Africans and Europeans. The EDAR gene is responsible for the East Asian hair type and arose during the past 65,000 years, when early humans were migrating "Out of Africa" into Europe, then Asia. The distributions of these straight hair related alleles support a hypothesis that our human ancestors had developed curly hair compared to other primates. The straight hair found in East Asia and the Indo-European subgroups almost certainly developed independently of each other.

Evolutionary Advantages of Straight and Curly Hair

Multiple theories exist why human beings who had left Africa developed the straight hair phenotype. These include improved comfort whilst hunting, improved UV light absorption for vitamin D production, and healthy bone development and sexual selection. A further theory is that human hair was reduced in response to parasite infestation wherein human nakedness is based on the principle that a hairless primate would carry fewer parasites. It may be that the ability to grow long, straight, densely packed hair provides an evolutionary advantage in cold climate and a distinct disadvantage in a hot climate, when compared to loosely packed, spongy, closely cropped hair.

Whatever the evolutionary pressure, straight hair presumably provided some biological advantage for hair health but only in humans who had left Africa. The persistence of curly hair throughout sub-equatorial Africa despite greater genetic diversity than in the rest of the world suggests that this phenotype has an evolutionary advantage. This is reinforced by this phenotype existing in peoples living at the Equator who have recent Asian lineages.

The current varied phenotypes of humans and their hair around the world may be explained by both genetics and the adaptations which occurred after the first migrations (diaspora) of modern humans out of Africa about 90,000 years ago. Hair morphology rose from the original tiny clans and as much as skin color, denotes our subgroup association.

Hair Color

Black and dark brown hair is the ubiquitous natural hair color in peoples of all regions. It accounts for over 90 % of all human hair color and is characterized by very high levels of the dark pigment eumelanin. Blond hair frequency is reported as 1.8 % on a worldwide basis.

There is no comparable data for red hair but in the areas of obvious frequency (the fringes of Western and Eastern Europe) it is at a maximum 10 % in Scotland (population 5 million) although 35 % of the population carry the recessive gene. Of redheads 80 % have the melanocortin 1 receptor gene anomaly which occurred between 20,000 and 100,000 years ago.

Blond hair is characterized by low levels of the dark pigment eumelanin and higher levels of the pale pigment pheomelanin, the dominant pigment of red hair. Shades range from light brown to pale blond.

Natural lighter hair colors occur most often in Europe and less frequently in other areas and is the result of a genetic mutation that resulted in blond hair in Europe has been isolated to about 11,000 years ago during the last ice age and became the dominant color about 3000 years ago. High frequencies of light hair in northern latitudes are a result of the light skin adaptation to lower levels of sunlight, which reduces the prevalence of rickets caused by vitamin D deficiency. The darker pigmentation at higher latitudes in certain ethnic groups such as the Inuit is explained by a greater proportion of Vitamin D rich seafood in their diet.

Modern Lithuania has the highest percentage of people with blonde hair. Bleaching of hair to mimic blonde is common, especially among women. Bleached blond can be distinguished from natural blond hair by exposing it to ultraviolet light, as heavily bleached hair will glow, while natural blonde hair will not.

Gray Hair

Blond hair is the result of having little pigmentation in the hair strand. Grey hair occurs when melanin production decreases or stops, while poliosis, typically in spots is hair (and often the skin to which the hair is attached to) that never possessed melanin at all in the first place, or ceased for natural genetic reasons, generally in the first years of life.

The advent of high quality hair dyes has resulted in an explosion of color changing across the world. These processes have a significant impact on hair health (see Chap. 3).

The Physical Properties of Hair

Hair can be stretched, bent, and curled. It can absorb moisture or lose it. Its behavior can alter when it is wetted or when brushed.

Understanding these properties is important for coping with hair of different phenotypes and under different circumstances. It is especially important for the hair stylist who has to decide on achievable styles, desired processing, and, most importantly, continuing hair care regimes for clients.

Of the many properties of the hair shaft—the ability to regulate moisture content (or not) is one of the most profound for the concept of maintenance of hair health. The loss of control is visible on the streets of every major city. Such is the extent of this self-inflicted disorder the term *chronic hair dehydration* has been coined (Fig. 1.31).

Particularly for over-processed hair (see Chap. 3) the moisture content of hair is greater when the atmosphere is moist and humid, and less when the air is dry. The reason why hair "collapses" in hot, humid atmospheres is summed up by:

Heat and humidity:

- more moisture
- less static electricity
- collapse or poof

In dry conditions:

- less moisture
- more static electricity
- more volume (body)

Furthermore, when hair is wet, the cortex swells and the edges of the cuticle scales tend to lift. Consequently, there is more friction but no greater static charge on wet hair than on dry.

This can lead to matting and tangling developing during over-vigorous shampooing.

Porosity

Technically, porosity refers to the measure of empty spaces in a material, in this case the hair shaft, and can be expressed as a percentage between 0 and 100 %.

In reality porosity refers to the hair's ability, or inability, to absorb water or chemicals through the

Hair: The Cosmetic Aspects

Fig. 1.31 (**a–c**) Repeated chemical processing leads to chronic hair dehydration

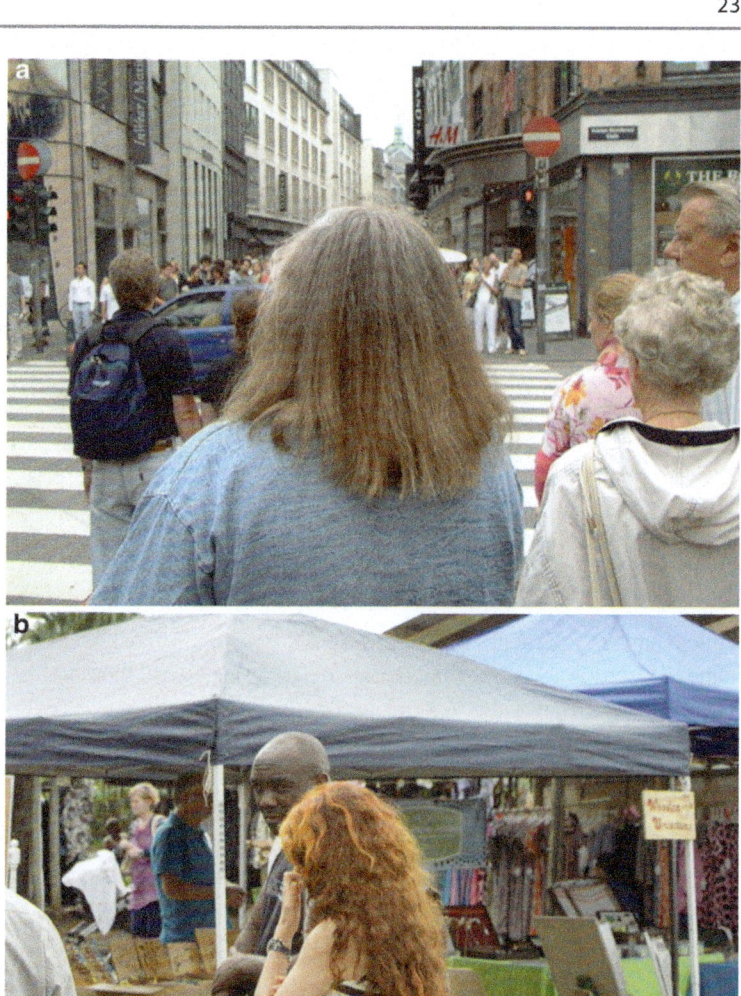
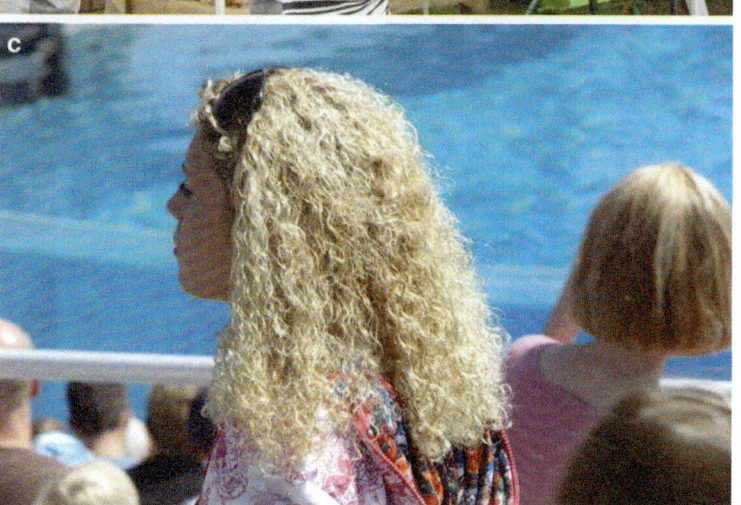

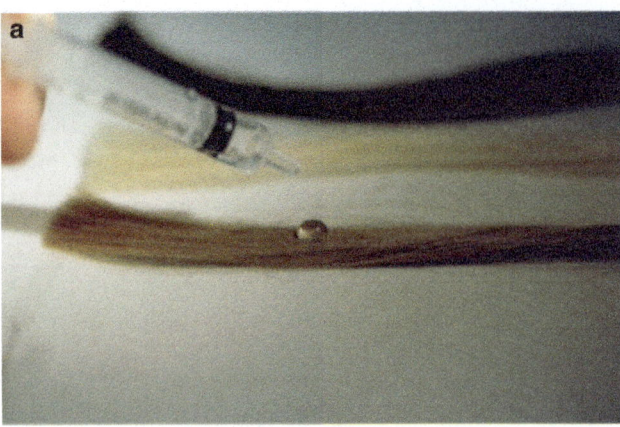 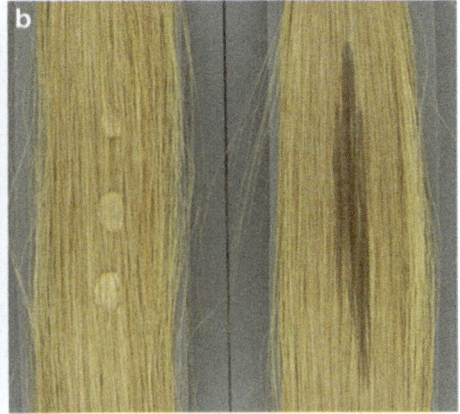

Fig. 1.32 A simple test of the porosity (or not) of a hair shaft. (**a**) A drop of water placed on the virgin hair does not soak in as the f-layer and cuticle are intact. (**b**) Bleached hair is highly porous and water is immediately absorbed

cuticle and into the mass of the cortex. All hair is naturally porous and somewhat permeable to water but intact hair resists this natural process via the restraining effect of the cuticle and particular, the f-layer. In a normal, undamaged hair shaft, the rate at which water can enter or exit out of the cortex is slow. However, hair can absorb up to 200 % of its weight in water, most commonly after perming when the f-layer has been removed, the cuticle is essentially "wide open" and the keratins in the cortex have been compromised (see Chap. 3).

Over-porous hair is dry, and tends to develop split ends. The damaged cuticle is fragile, and the damage worsens with time and repeated processing. The greater the damage, the more the cortex swells with water whenever the hair is washed and the more water it loses when it dries.

A simple test of the porosity of the hair is demonstrated by placing a drop of water on a hair tress which is undamaged and one which has been repeatedly processed. On the undamaged hair the water droplet retains its shape due to the intact cuticle. On the damaged hair, it is rapidly absorbed (Fig. 1.32).

Elasticity

This is an important property of hair. Due to its elasticity, hair can resist forces that could change its shape, volume, or length and allowing it to return to its original form without damage.

When healthy hair is wetted and stretched, it can increase in length by up to 30 % and still return to its original length when dried. Stretching it in excess of 30 % tends to damage resulting in permanent lengthening and even breaking.

The elasticity of hair depends on the long keratin fibers in the cortex. Chemical treatments such as perming and bleaching can alter the cortex after repeated damage and affect hair's elasticity. Hair with poor elasticity will stretch only to a limited extent. It will not curl, it will break easily when it is groomed, and it cannot be permed satisfactorily.

Both natural sunlight and artificial ultraviolet light break down keratin in the hair and damage its elasticity in the same way that bleaching does, though to a much lesser degree.

The elastic properties of both wet and dry hair are related to the diameter of the hair shaft. The thicker the hair, the more it will tend to resist stretching.

The graph below illustrates the percentage stretching of wet and dry hair tresses (Fig. 1.33).

Static Electricity

When dry hair is rubbed, as it is whenever it is brushed or combed, static electric charge builds up on the hairs. This is especially noticeable in hot, dry weather. The charges tend to repel neighboring hairs and as a result charged hairs can

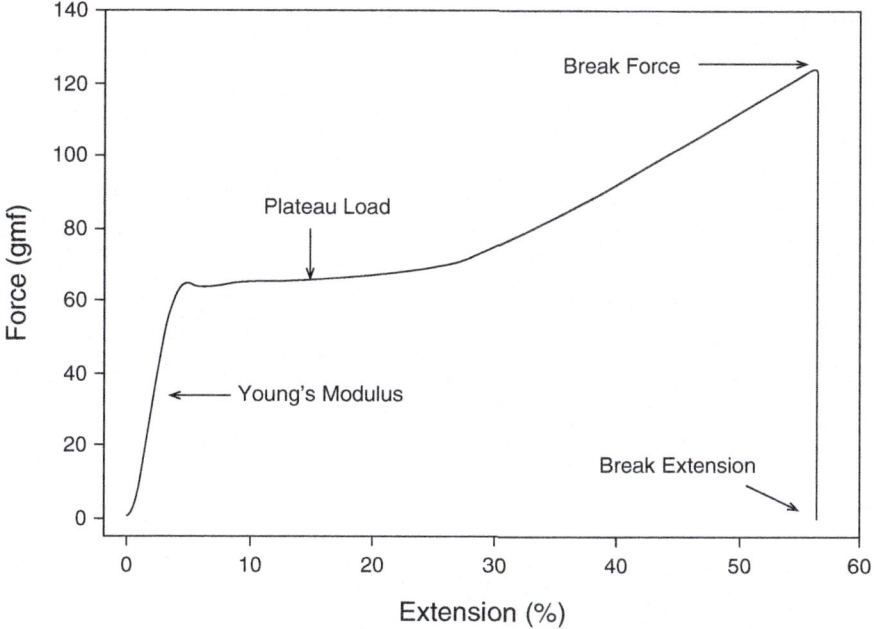

Fig. 1.33 Wet and dry stress strain for wet and dry hair

never lie smoothly against each other. The result is "fly away" hair, which stands out from the head and looks unmanageable.

Texture

Much of the attraction of a beautiful head of hair lies in its texture, or feel which is dependent on several parameters. Primarily it is due to the average diameter of the individual hairs. The larger the hair diameter, the coarser it will feel (Fig. 1.34).

Secondly, is natural variation—some hair feels hard and others soft, some silky and others wiry. The reasons underlying these differences are still a matter for scientific conjecture.

Thirdly, the texture is affected by the degree of weathering of the hair. See Chap. 2. If hair is processed too many times the cuticle scales may never return to their original tightness and the protection they once offered is lost. The cuticle can also be damaged in the same way by too much blow drying, curling irons that are too hot, and the effects of wind and sun. The hair becomes increasingly porous, and water can then pass in and out of the cortex.

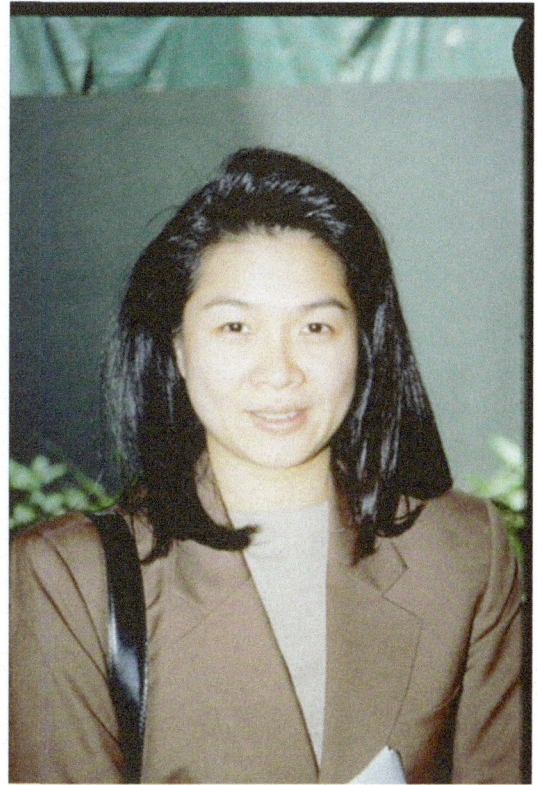

Fig. 1.34 Bangkok – hair—with large diameter and straight, with a powerful texture

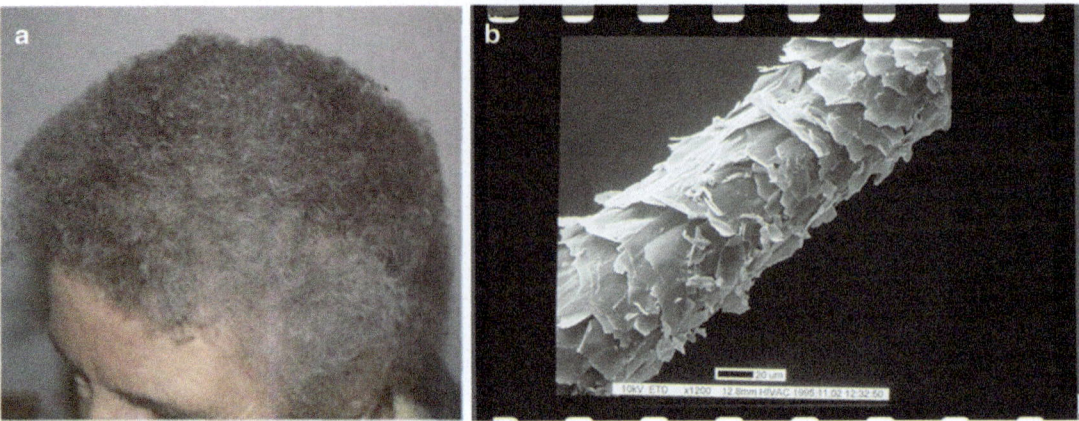

Fig. 1.35 (**a**) In later life this lady's hair has become naturally shorter and thinner, with less body; perming, which she has chosen as a way of correcting this, has resulted in dryness and loss of texture. (**b**) Damage to the cuticle, caused by over-perming, will alter the texture of the hair

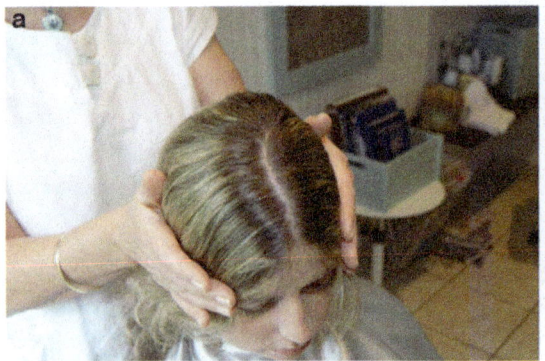
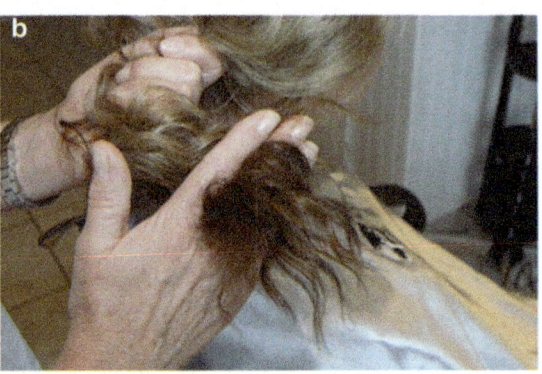

Fig. 1.36 The difference from (**a**) roots to (**b**) tip. As a dead structure, the hair shaft nevertheless records the damage inflicted on it. This so-called "Record of the hair" is important in assessing when, how, and where damage was inflicted

Finally, hair texture is affected by what has been applied to it. Repeated lavish applications of hair spray gives hair a different feel from that of hair that has been freshly washed and conditioned. Conditioners make hair feel soft and smooth. Conditioners that contain silicones even give a slightly different feel from those that don't (most manufacturers now employ silicones into conditioners as they protect the hair cuticle). Contrary to popular belief, this altered feel is not a sign of build-up (Fig. 1.35).

The Concept of Root to Tip

Newly emerging hair has properties that are different from those of the hair tips. The last few inches of long hair, particularly the last 4 inches and the tip, has typically undergone several hundred washes, the application of hot styling implements, and other cosmetic procedures such as bleaching, permanent coloring, and perming in addition to normal exposure to the environment. It would be a miraculous material not to show changes, the cumulative effects of the above is termed weathering.

As a dead structure, the hair shaft nevertheless records the damage inflicted on it. This so-called "Record of the hair" is important in assessing when, how, and where damage was inflicted. As Dr Steven Shiel has stated "the hair never forgets- everything that ever happened is there for all to see."

Hair also harbors chemicals (legal or otherwise) which have been ingested and again can provide a forensic record along its length (Fig. 1.36).

Previously this damage could only be assessed with the naked eye and the touch or the electron micrograph (EMG) (Fig. 1.37).

Recently cosmetic scientists have been able to record damage by assessment of the degradation of protein content and environmental metals. This they are able to do long before the gross consequences of damage become visible.

Hair care and hair care products are designed to cleanse and render the hair in a fit state for ease of grooming. The range of human hair—long and straight to short and intensely curled—challenges the product formulator. The degree of damage inflicted on hair raises that challenge to greater heights (Figs. 1.38 and 1.39).

In the next chapter we explore the reality of healthy hair.

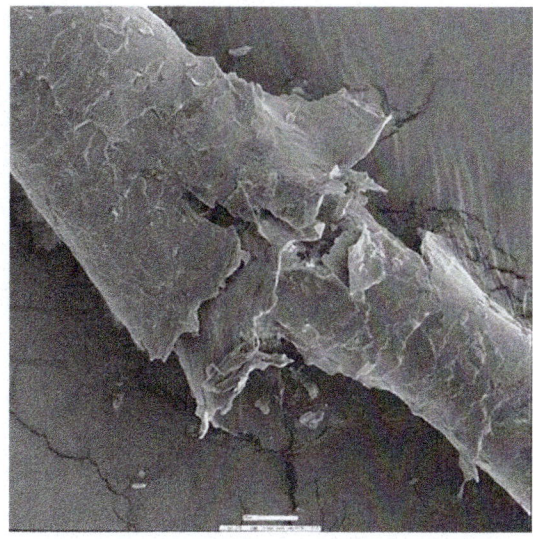

Fig. 1.37 Almost complete fracture of the hair shaft under the electron micrograph

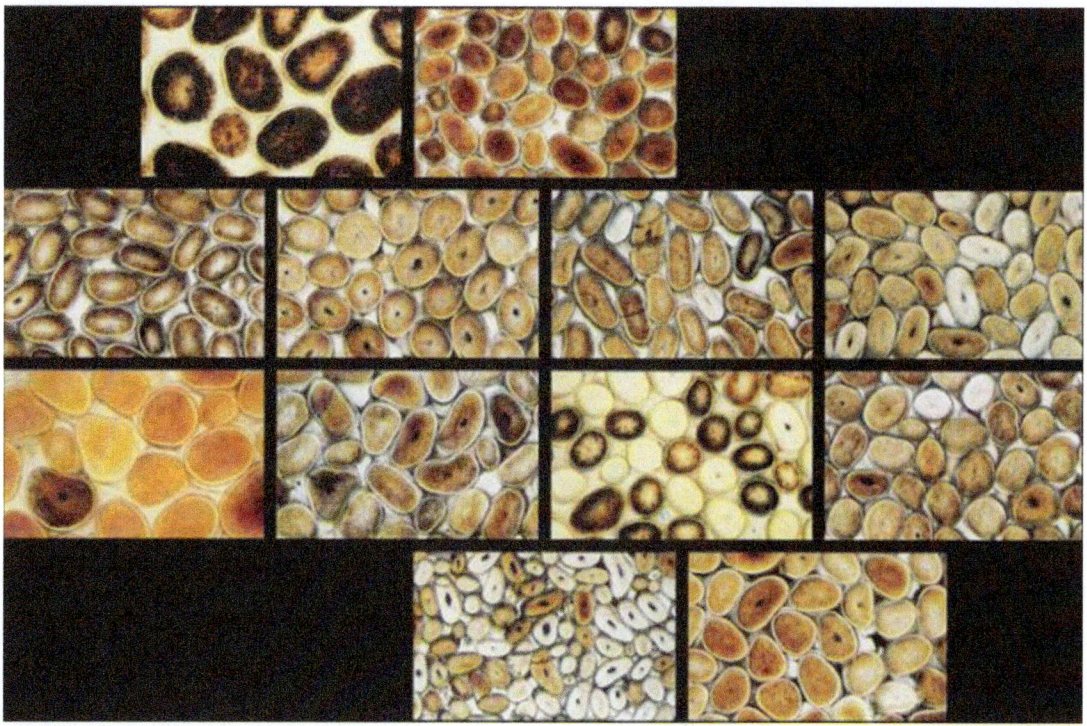

Fig. 1.38 Images illustrating hair shape, color, and size variations on single heads

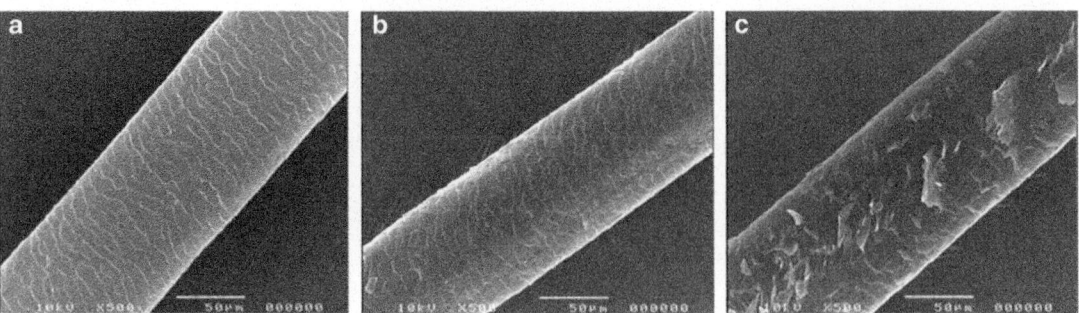

Fig. 1.39 (a–c) SEM images of root, mid and tips of women with 30 cm length hair illustrating change in hair structure

Reference

1. Birch PM, Messenger A. Bad hair days – scalp sebum excretion and the menstrual cycle. J Cosmet Dermatol. 2004, 2 (3–40), 190–194.

Further Reading

Blume-Peytavi U, Tosti A, Whiting D, Trueb R. Hair growth & disorders. Springer; 2008.

McMichael A, Hordinsky MK. Hair & scalp diseases. Informa; 2008.

Root-to-Tip Hair Health

Introduction

Human hair is only displayed in any volume on the head for good evolutionary reasons. The faces of our hunter-gatherer forebears would not have been easily visible across the open veldt, plain, or tundra to prospective enemies, friends, or potential mates. Nor indeed, in subsequent generations, is it easily seen across the darkened nightclub floor. It is the appearance of scalp hair that, in conjunction with body form, is the immediate and key component of attraction. At a distance, or from behind, the quality of a person's hair may imply an age (youth, health, and fecundity) not reinforced by facial markers (Fig. 2.1a–c).

Conversely, facial beauty may be marred or distracted from by unkempt and/or unhealthy hair. In the twenty-first century "health" is synonymous with "youth." In many cultures, this latter asset is not only admired but also worshiped. The desire to look younger than one's chronological age is driven by remorseless real or perceived social pressures.

The explosion in plastic surgery and bleaching blonde is further testimony to this desire for youth. An inevitable corollary to this desire is that hair has never been under such "attack." Repeated chemical and physical processing and so-called "keratin" hair treatments have had significant consequences for hair health. Fortunately, unlike skin, hair can regrow after the worst disasters.

A whole industry has been founded on hair care, and the world's most successful hair care brand has identified that the concept of "hair health" as exemplified by shine, feel, and manageability is critically important to millions of women. Yet a promenade down any street today reveals the extent of "unhealthy" hair.

In the previous chapter we described the structure of normal human hair. In this chapter we explore the concept of "hair health" and its importance to all women. This chapter seeks to define and demonstrate these signs of hair health and by doing so, allow women to more easily make a judgmental assessment of their own hair.

These questions are considered with reference to different hair phenotypes and the impact on hair health for women as they chronologically age.

The advent of investigative tools such as proteomics and genomics has allowed hair care scientists to identify and, more importantly, quantify, what constitutes "healthy" hair. These breakthroughs have allowed a radical shift in the design and development of hair care products to protect and maintain hair health.

Healthy Hair

Hair is seldom healthier than in childhood since, at this stage, it is relatively undamaged by the host. It illustrates the key signs of health—shine, feel, and an almost magical vitality related to its anatomical and physiological integrity (Fig. 2.2).

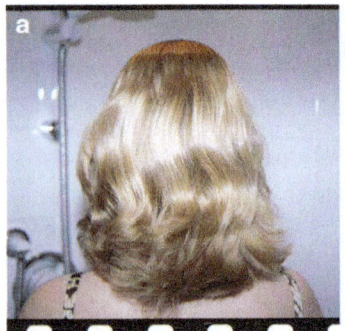 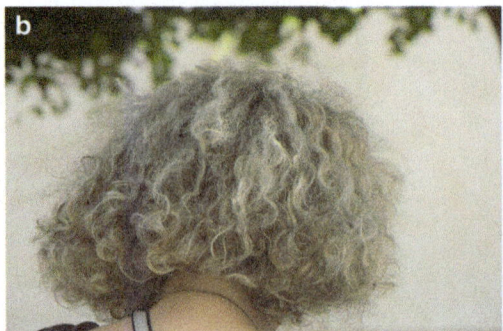 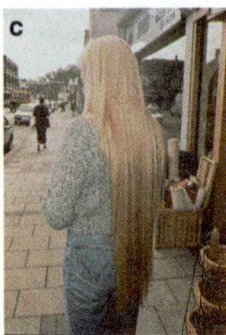

Fig. 2.1 From behind, hair may imply age and health which the facial features may or may not reinforce: (**a**) age 17; (**b**) age 34; and (**c**) age 45

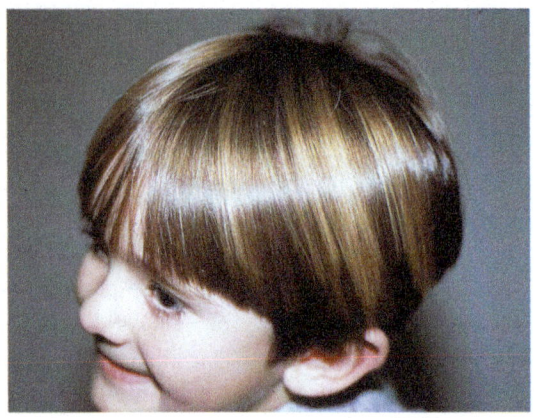

Fig. 2.2 Beautiful hair. This young boy's hair displays a massive shine band and magical vitality. Interestingly, he also displays an inherited mosaicism—with multiple bands of natural pigment

A technical description of healthy hair has been proposed as "shiny hair with a smooth texture and clean-cut ends or tapered tips and well moisturized" (more likely "not dry") [1]. This, of course, does not take into account the significant differences in the phenotypes of hair around the world and the expectation of what can be achieved. Most notably, women of African descent have hair which, due to its phenotype, is naturally more prone to dryness and almost impossible without chemical or heat intervention.

This chapter will describe these attributes in more detail and explore how women around the world perceive hair health.

Women's Perception of Hair Health

Day-to-day judgment of one's hair status is invariably based on a rapid assessment of the overall appearance and feel and includes both its manageability and ability to hold a style, particularly in a humid or variable climate.

Women's perception of hair health has been assessed by extensive consumer research. For those wishing to develop products, a critical question is whether women do, indeed, have a view as to whether their hair is essentially healthy or damaged.

In a study conducted by P&G with women from European and Oriental hair phenotypes (US, UK, Japan, China, Mexico) and a study conducted with women from African phenotypes (Brazil, Nigeria, South Africa) the data showed that the majority of women consider themselves to have some level of hair damage, and in many regions this is more than 80 %. The exception is in Nigeria and South Africa, but more detailed research indicated these women have concerns about hair breakage and dryness but do not associate this directly with hair damage. From the same studies, approximately 50 % of respondents stated they were either extremely concerned or very concerned about their hair health, and less than 5 % of women were not at all concerned, suggesting that not only is lack of hair health (essentially hair damage) a global reality, but is also of major concern.

The term "healthy hair" is vague and covers a multitude of different signals. Graphic 1 shows

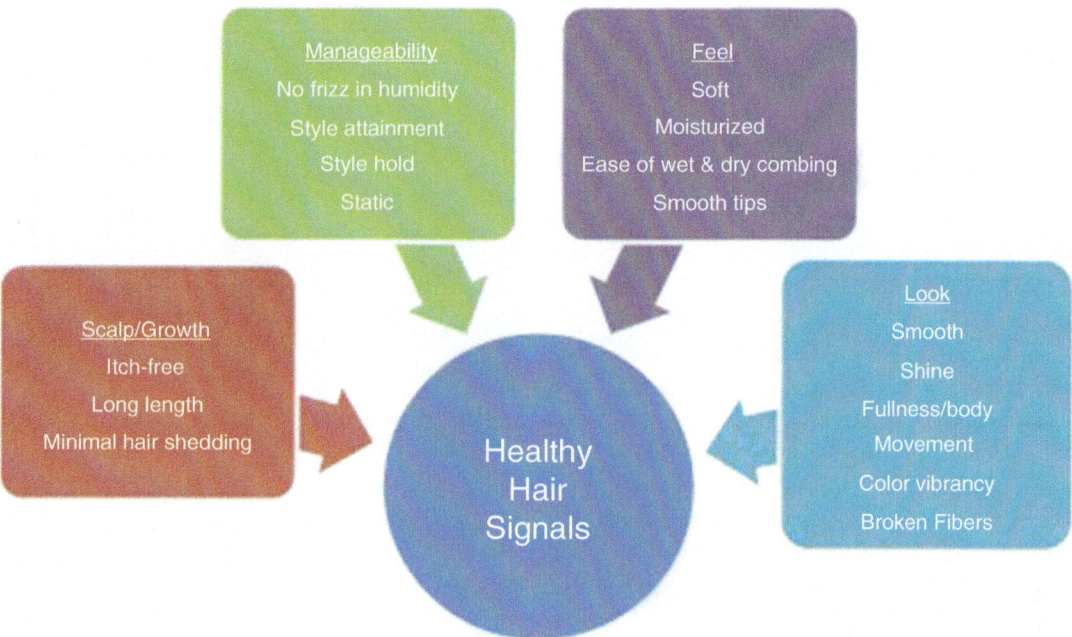

Fig. 2.3 Healthy hair signals

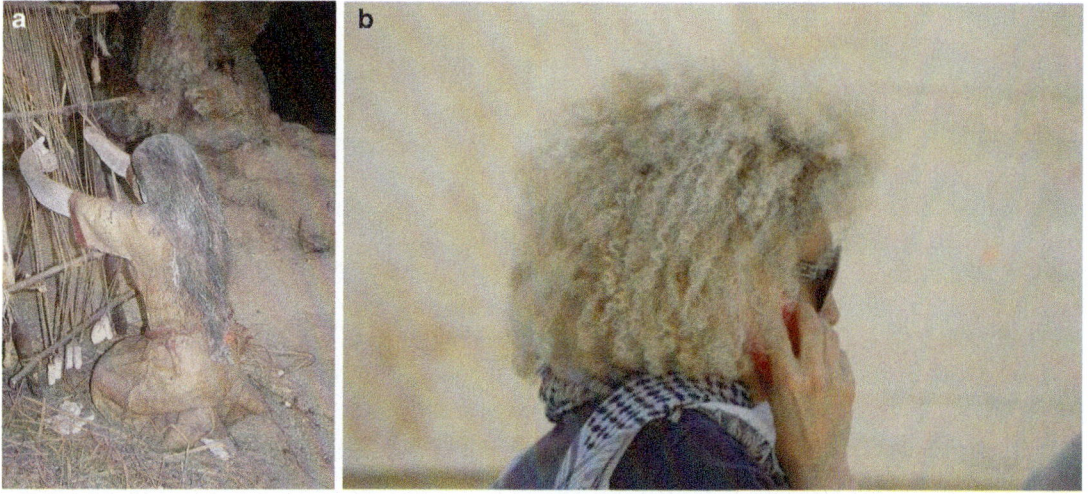

Fig. 2.4 Bad hair days (**a**) circa 4000 years BC—courtesy of Topkapi Museum, Istanbul; and (**b**) in Italy 2014

a schematic illustration of the common answers given by women globally to the question "How do you know if your hair is healthy?" (Fig. 2.3).

In reality the final assessment of the health of any one head of hair will be a combination of many factors and different senses (touch, look, sound). The signals may also vary from day to day depending on whether the respondent is experiencing a host of subliminal influences (mood, hormone status) and frank physical influences such as weather and humidity. All may be impactful in a "bad hair" day (Fig. 2.4a, b).

Of these many parameters there are five top indicators of hair health that are important to the majority of women globally. These are

1. shine
2. no damaged tips/split ends
3. smoothness/no frizz
4. desired volume
5. no breakage/strength

There are, as might be expected, some global differences in the relative importance of these factors. Thirty percent of Caucasian women tend to rate inability to create the right volume, i.e., the style is too flat and limp, as the most important signal of damage. This is less of an issue for Oriental and women of African descent (<10 %). The relative importance also varies with style, for example, breakage and damaged tips tend to be a more important signal for women with longer hair.

Of these five parameters of hair health it is incumbent to explore the technical reasons why they are such manifest indicators.

Sign 1: Shine

Shine is the single most important signal of healthy hair for many women. It is de facto the main area where they would like to see improvement in their appearance. In women's minds, healthy hair has natural sheen and luster, is bright, and has vitality (Figs. 2.5 and 2.6).

In the same manner as healthy hair is seen as "youthful," hair without shine due to overprocessing can mimic chronological aging and sends confusing signals (Fig. 2.7).

Shine is not merely judged by a reflection in a mirror, but by other subliminal criteria. Inquiry regarding shine invariably precipitates touching and running of the fingers through the subject's hair. If hair feels smooth and aligned, the perception of shine may be greater.

Oddly, abnormal levels of shine may occur when products such as heavy oils and some serums are used. These products can give hair an oily or greasy appearance, and the hair may feel

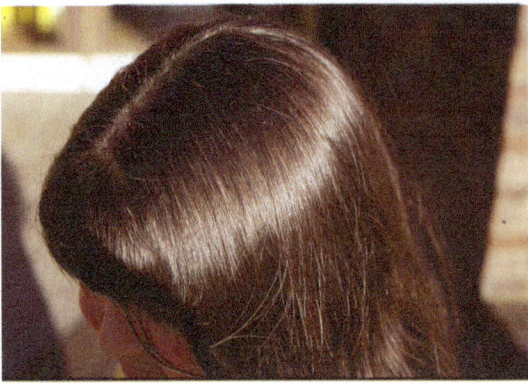

Fig. 2.5 In many women's minds, healthy hair has natural sheen and luster, is bright, and has vitality

weighed down, which leads to a negative shine perception (Fig. 2.8).

Physical Aspects of Shine

Shine is generated by light reflection from a smooth and intact surface of the hair shaft into the observer's eye. Shine perception is a combination of hair alignment, specular, chroma, and diffuse reflection components. It is strongly dependent on hair color, as this determines the level of chroma reflection present.

Specular shine is a mirror-like reflection of light from a surface in which light from a single incoming direction is reflected into a single outgoing direction. This is typical of hair in which the cuticle is undisturbed (Fig. 2.9).

Diffuse reflection is due to incoming light being reflected in a broad range of directions, and is common from hair in which the cuticle is severely disrupted. The cuticle is of particular importance for light scattering, since it forms the interface between the fiber and the air (Fig. 2.10).

Chroma reflection is the quality of color that embraces both hue and saturation (black and white have no hues). The chroma of hair reveals the color information that is locked inside the hair fiber. It is an area found at the outer parts of the shine band and integrates shine and color information. The chroma band is based on partial light absorption by pigments and reflection of the remaining light, and is a measure for healthy looking hair (Figs. 2.11 and 2.12).

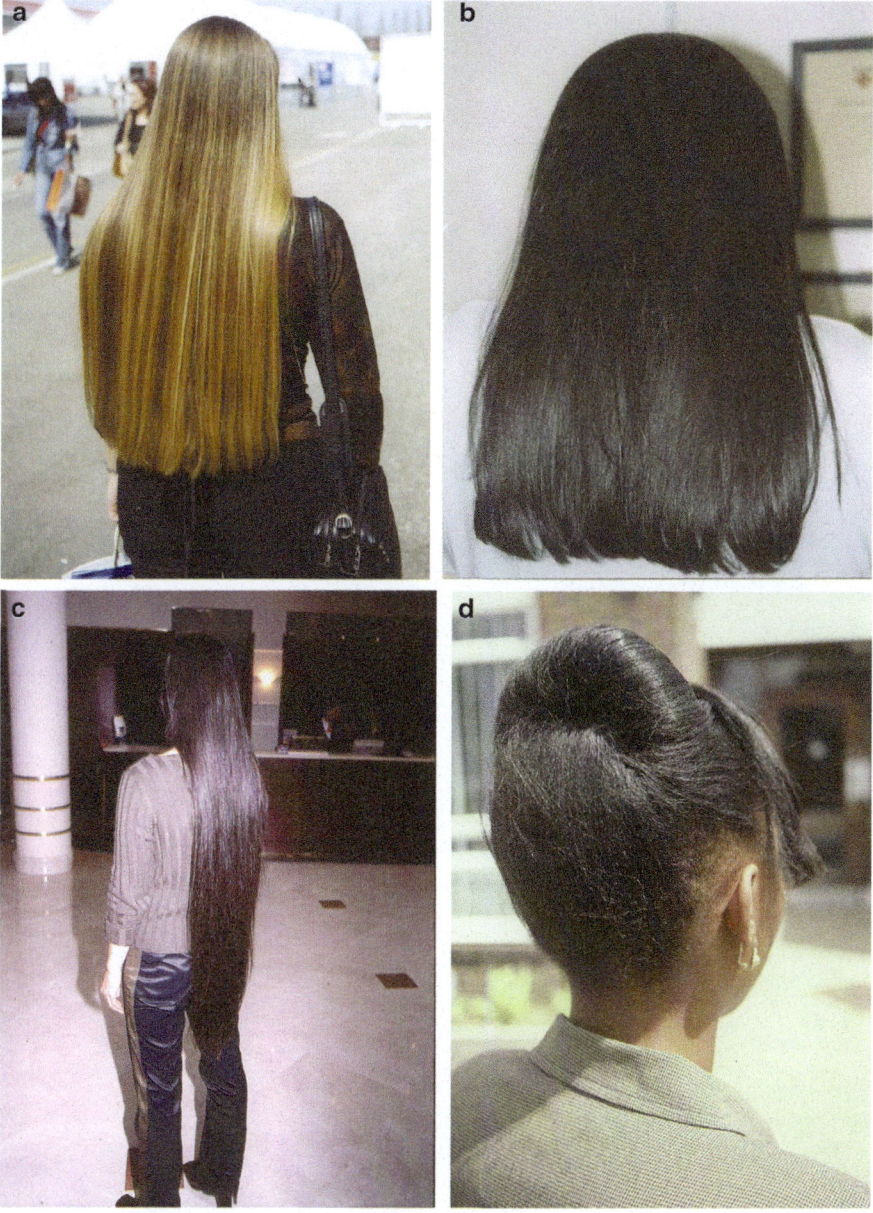

Fig. 2.6 Regardless of whether hair origin is (**a**) Continental Europe, (**b**) India, (**c**) China, or (**d**) South Africa (relaxed), shine is regarded as a key marker of hair health

The **shine band** is the area of hair that reflects the majority of light toward the viewer's eyes and is a unique characteristic of natural hair. It consists of reflection from the front and the back of the hair as well as diffuse reflection from the individual hair fibers.

The cuticle acts as a mirror that reflects a certain ratio of light—the higher the number of layers, the higher the ratio of the reflected light and the more intense the shine. The shine band analysis is used as a test method to assess the healthy look of hair (Fig. 2.13a, b).

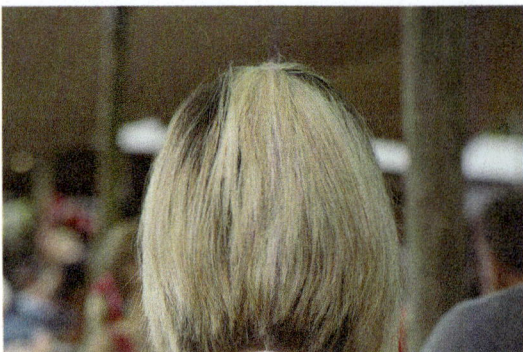

Fig. 2.7 Hair without shine can be aging

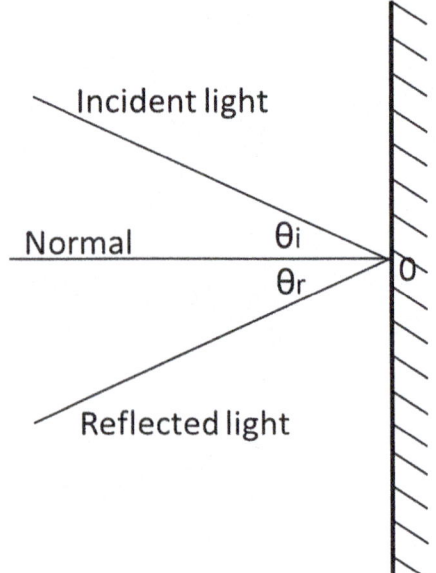

Fig. 2.9 Specular shine is a mirror-like reflection of light from a surface in which light from a single incoming direction is reflected into a single outgoing direction

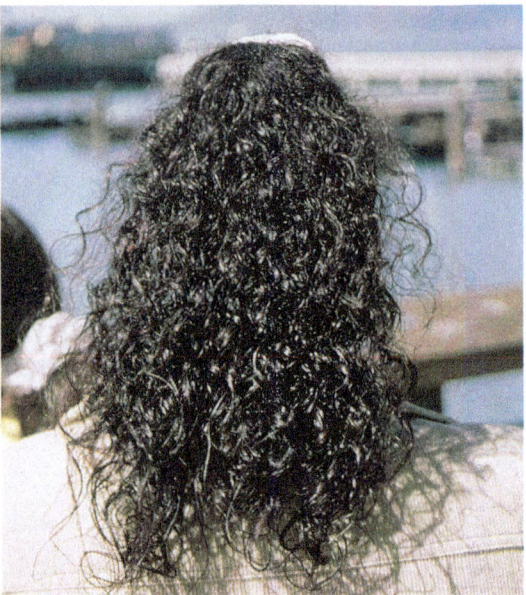

Fig. 2.8 Abnormal levels of shine may occur when products such as heavy oils and some serums are used

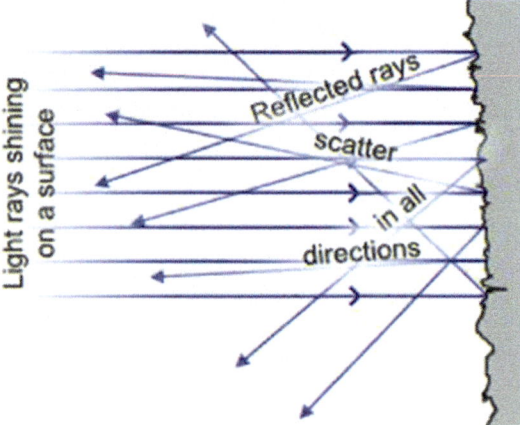

Fig. 2.10 Diffuse reflection is where incoming light is reflected in a broad range of directions, and is common from hair in which the cuticle is severely disrupted

Shine and Curls

Achieving shine from curls is a challenge since factors such as the structure of the hair, alignment problems, sebum build-up, accumulated styling products, damage from heat or chemicals, dirt, and pollution all interfere with reflection. If the hair shaft is damaged and the cuticle is roughened, light will not reflect back strongly, since it is diffused (Fig. 2.14).

Of all hair types, African hair is the most difficult on which to produce a shine. The flattened nature of the hair shaft and the intense curl defeats specular reflection and all the light is diffused, creating a "matte" effect. Many women with African hair now relax and straighten it and achieve better alignment, which improves reflection. However, this phenotype still requires a substantial moisturizing product and often, oil-based formulations to create significant shine (Figs. 2.15 and 2.16).

Healthy Hair

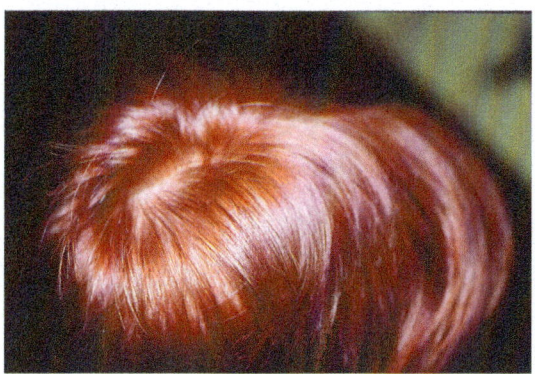

Fig. 2.11 The chroma of hair reveals the color information that is locked inside the hair fiber

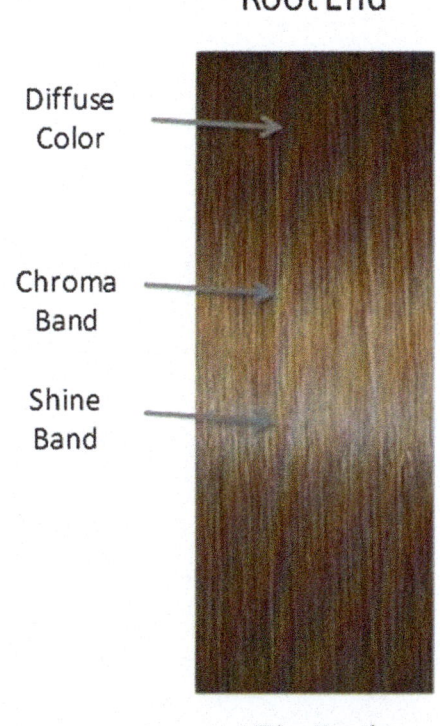

Fig. 2.12 Color, chroma, and shine bands from root to tip

Styling, Color, and Shine

Styling and color can enhance shine. Defined curls produce more shine than a mass of small curls because of the nature of the eye. To achieve this with curly or wavy hair, styling the hair in sections to create bigger curls is advisable. In the hands of an expert colorist, color treatments may enhance shine, even bearing in mind the inherent structural changes to the hair shaft, since it intensifies the color inside the cortex and enhances the chroma element. When light enters and is reflected, the shine appears more intense. The darker the color, the more intense the shine bands appear due to the contrast between the chroma band and the color.

As hair loses its pigment and turns gray, diffuse light scattering increases, making the hair appear less shiny. This contributes to the perception that aging hair is less healthy, along with other changes such as decreased diameter and density.

The Psychological Aspects of Shine

The International Congress and Symposium Series published in 2008 "Assessment of Hair Quality Using Eye-Tracking Technology," which was sponsored by an educational grant from P&G [2]. Naive observers were presented with computer images of women with different types of hair (messy, frizzy, straight, curly, etc.) and laser technology mounted in an eye-tracker device—originally developed for fighter jet pilots—tracked how much time they spent looking at different elements on the computer screen (for further details see Chap. 3).

Surprisingly, shiny hair, although it was the first reference point, was only transiently so. The data determined that the eye moves rapidly on to the face. A greater time was spent looking at dull and frizzy hair. The conclusion drawn is that shine is an almost subliminal reassurance of health, and thus the eyes move on to the key target—the face. Frizzy and unkempt hair is not only a distraction, but is also assessed and designated as unhealthy and less attractive.

Shine and Weathering

Shine inevitably decreases with the weathering (see Chap. 3) which occurs from root to tip due to the cumulative impact of the environment and self-inflicted physical and chemical damage over time (Fig. 2.17).

For the cosmetic chemist who is formulating hair-care products, multiple measures and metrics

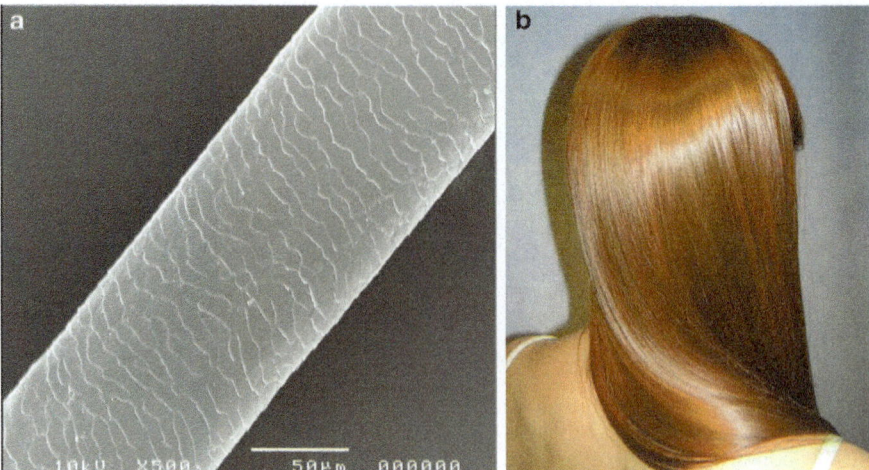

Fig. 2.13 (**a**) The cuticle is of particular importance for light scattering, since it forms the interface between the fiber and the air. (**b**) A prominent shine band with strong chroma reflection. The shine of hair reveals information about the surface properties of hair

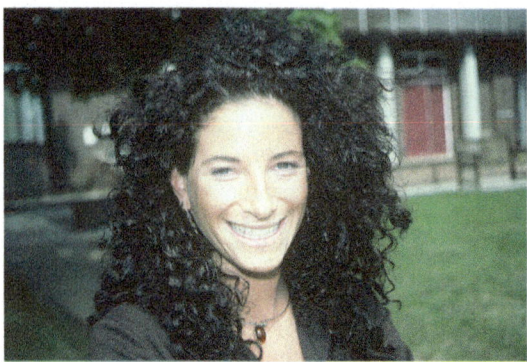

Fig. 2.14 Getting curls to shine may be a challenge, since hair structure, alignment problems, sebum build-up, accumulated styling products, damage from heat or chemicals, dirt, and pollution all can interfere with shine

are required to quantify the total effect of products and damage prevention on shine (see Chap. 5).

Shampoos provide shine by cleaning the hair surface of sebum, dirt, and product deposits. Conditioners provide shine by increasing lubricity of hair, making it easier to align fibers. Hair color provides shine by increasing background

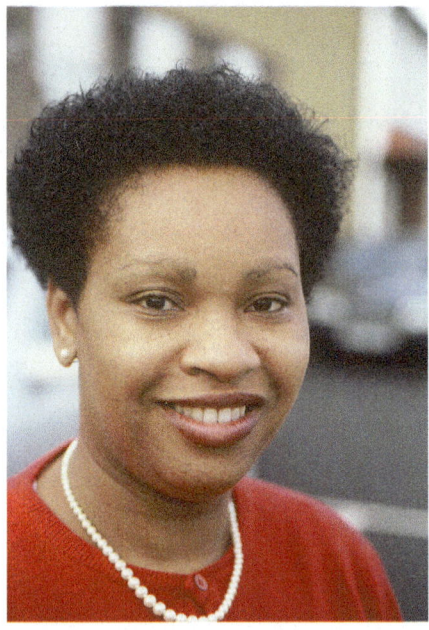

Fig. 2.15 The flattened nature of the African hair shaft and the intense curl defeats specular reflection, and the majority of light is diffused, creating a "matte" effect. This lady relaxes her hair and then has it re-fixed with a looser curl

Healthy Hair

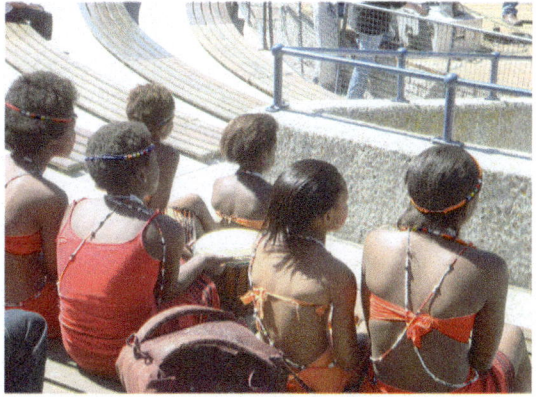

Fig. 2.16 The whole gamut of hair types in young African women (Cape Town). Note the relaxed hair has far greater shine due to alignment and apparent moisturization, possibly due to the use of oils

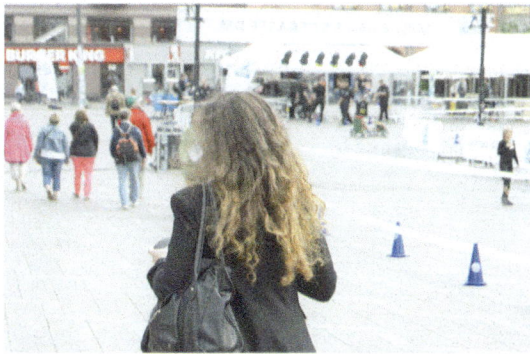

Fig. 2.17 Weathering from root to tip. The impact of the environment and self-inflicted physical and chemical damage increases over time, and is most evident by the lack of shine

contrast and chroma reflection of hair. Dark hair is often perceived as having maximum shine vs. lighter shades, due to the higher contrast between the bright shine band and the background hair color (Fig. 2.18a, b).

Shine Summary

Shine is a primary indicator of hair health.

- Shine perception is comprised of hair alignment, specular, chroma, and diffuse reflection components.
- Shine decreases with weathering from root to tip.
- Shine decreases with chemical and physical damage.
- Shampoos provide shine by cleaning the hair surface of sebum, dirt, and product deposits.
- Conditioners provide shine by increasing lubricity of hair, making it easier to align fibers.
- Hair color provides shine by increasing background contrast and chroma reflection of hair.

Sign 2: Absence of Split Ends/Damaged Tips

The casual observer may see women feeling their tip ends by running fingers through their hair. In addition, those with longer hair will look at their tips for signs of broken, misaligned fibers and split ends. These signs are a direct measure of healthy hair and, if present, are an indicator that a trim is due.

Immediately after a haircut the hair tips will be aligned at the same length and with a flat end surface. Over time, as hair is exposed to washing and brushing, the ends become frayed and in some cases form split ends. In this case the cuticle has typically been removed and the cortical cells split into smaller fragments that travel up the hair length. At this stage the damage is visible to the naked eye (Fig. 2.19a–c).

Other signals of damaged tips include reduced ponytail length from hair mid-length to tip and slightly lighter tips. For those with straight, dark hair (e.g., women from India, China, Japan) the tips can appear browner than the mid-length and the roots. This color change is mainly driven by diffuse light scattering from the damaged tips (Fig. 2.20).

Tip hair is especially susceptible to breakage and physical abrasion because as hair is combed or brushed, this is where is where tangles are most likely to form. It also has experienced the most weathering, so is more likely to have split ends, which more easily tangle. Within the tangle, fibers are forced into close proximity with one another, and thus increased frictional forces will increase damage by abrading the cuticle

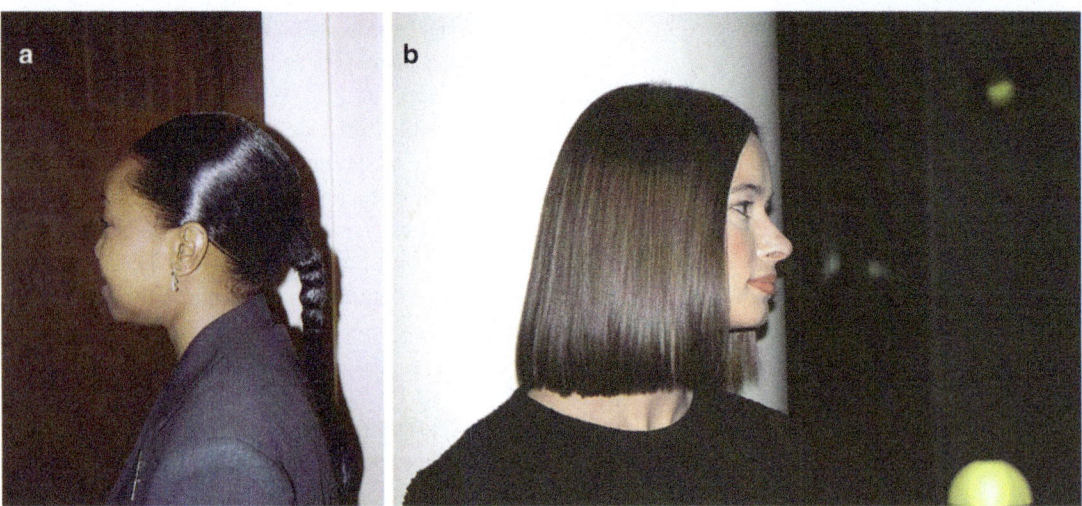

Fig. 2.18 (**a**) Dark hair is often perceived as having maximum shine vs. lighter brown or blonde hair, but (**b**) shine can also come from color variation, such as the highlights in this professionally colored and styled hair

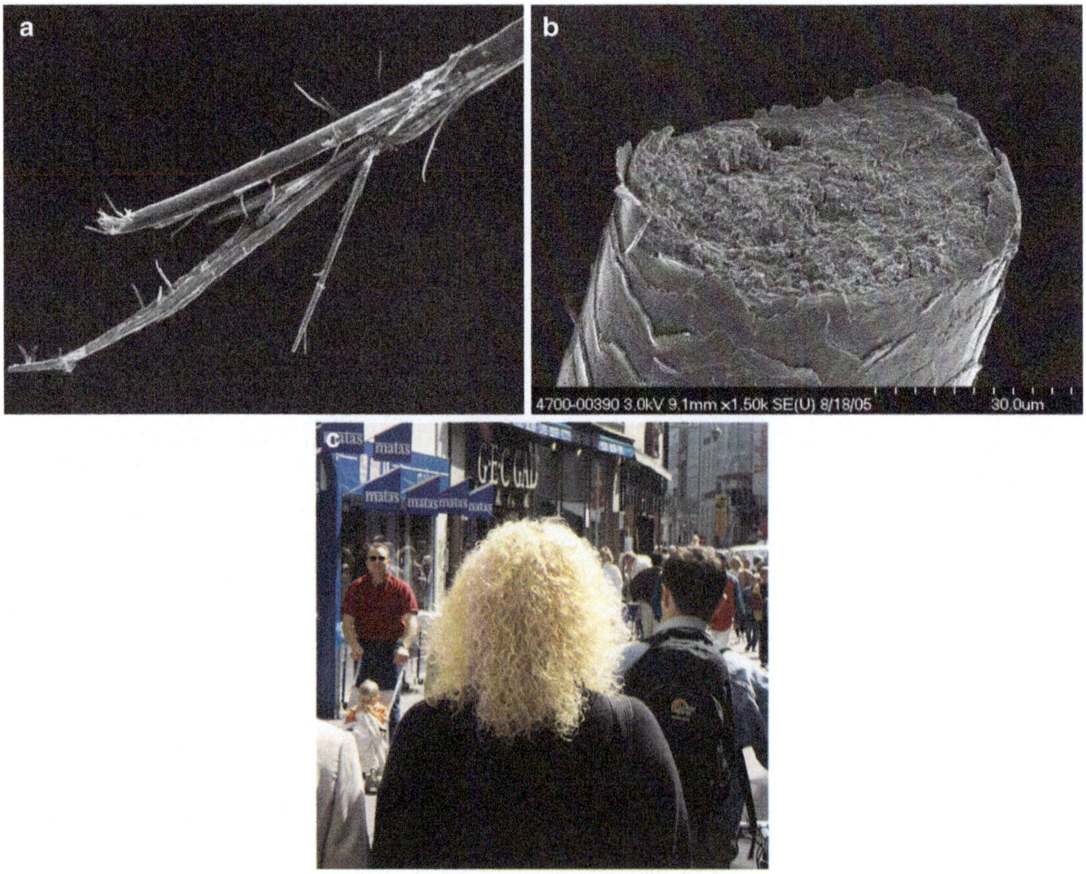

Fig. 2.19 (**a**) A typical split end—the only option at this stage is a trim; (**b**) showing end after trim; (**c**) damaged ends to the naked eye in over-processed hair

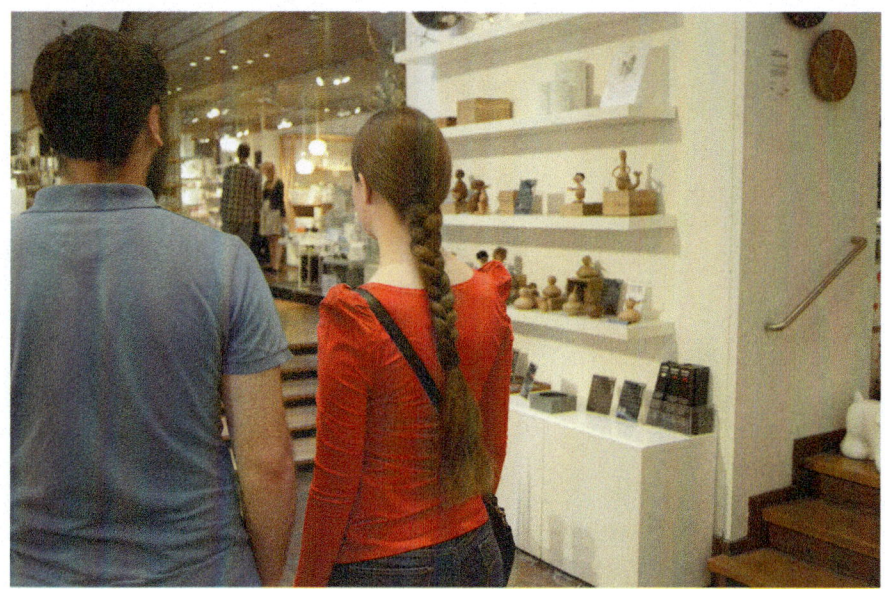

Fig. 2.20 Even in this young woman, the diffuse light from the tips of this otherwise powerful ponytail indicates damage

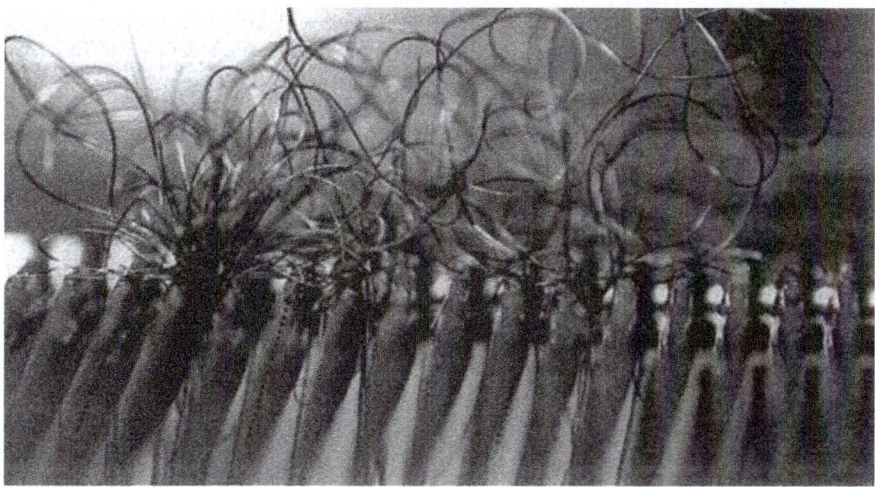

Fig. 2.21 Tangles formed in a comb

structure. In addition, these forces may be strong enough to form fractures and damage (Figs. 2.21 and 2.22).

Hair curvature is a very significant contributor to breakage and tip damage, as tangles and knots are much more likely to form in curly vs. straight hair. This tip breakage is a significant concern for women of African descent where the tight curl and twist of hair makes breakage from tangling during combing more common. Often damage can be seen to the cuticles on the outside of the curl where physical abrasion between fibers is higher (Fig. 2.23).

For straight hair, tangles and tip damage during wet combing is higher than during dry combing, but the opposite is true for curly hair. For straight hair it is friction between fibers that

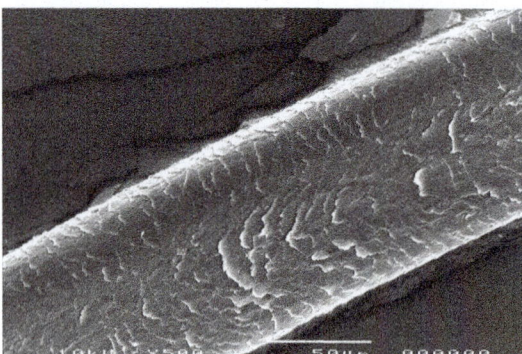

Fig. 2.22 Scanning Electron Microscope (SEM) image of combing damage to hair tips

dominates and the higher frictional forces of wet hair lead to more damage. For curly hair, curvature dominates and curvature is lower when hair is wet vs. dry so dry hair is more susceptible to tangles and tip damage.

Use of chemical treatments will also have a significant impact on broken fibers and damaged tips. This is caused by increased frictional forces from chemical removal of the hydrophilic lipid F-layer, creating a surface which has higher friction. These products can also weaken the inherent strength of hair, making it more brittle. For example, women who use chemical relaxing products to straighten hair often see very high tip damage.

Products such as conditioners are ideally suited to reducing this damage by providing lubrication to each fiber, allowing them to easily pass each other and reduce tangles and knots.

Sign 3: Smoothness/Frizz-Free

Absence of frizz is a key signal that hair is healthy, but how women describe frizz can vary widely according to hair type and style. One manifestation of frizz is small fibers sticking up at the parting line and fibers through the hair length that project away from the main body of hair. This type of frizz is more obvious for women with straight hair who are seeking a smooth look. These small fibers will also decrease hair shine and also negatively influence hair feel. Related to

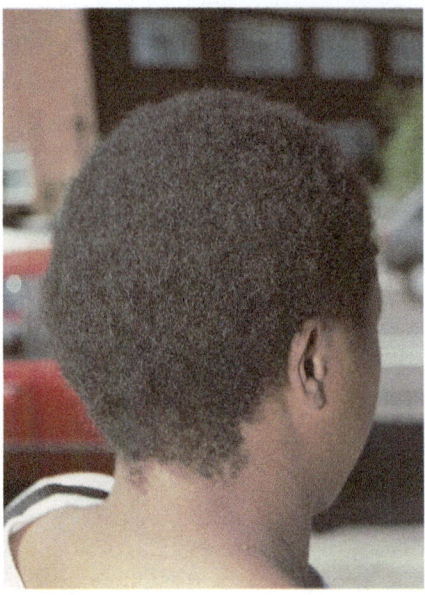

Fig. 2.23 Tip breakage is a significant concern for women of African descent where the tight curl and twist of hair makes breakage from tangling during combing more common

this can be a misalignment of tip hair, which is especially obvious when the tips are damaged. Cuticle loss and split ends mean hair does not lie in an aligned position and can be described as "frizzy" (Fig. 2.24).

Another manifestation of frizz is loss of alignment in hair, and is often described by women with wavy or curly hair. Instead of all fibers aligning in a controlled curl, each fiber has its own shape, leading to less curl and more frizz (Fig. 2.25a–d).

Frizz is often associated with weather conditions and, in particular, high humidity and high temperatures. Women may have achieved their desired style in the morning, but after a few hours of humidity exposure, the style is lost and has taken on the manifestations of frizz described above. The more uncontrollable the hair becomes in humidity (i.e., loss of alignment, shine, and style), the more hair is perceived as unhealthy.

The cause of humidity-created frizz is diffusion of water vapor inside hair. Hair at high humidity can take up 15–20 % of its own weight vs. fully dry hair, and the rate of uptake increases at higher temperatures. Hair is extremely

Healthy Hair

Fig. 2.24 Frizz in a straight hair style

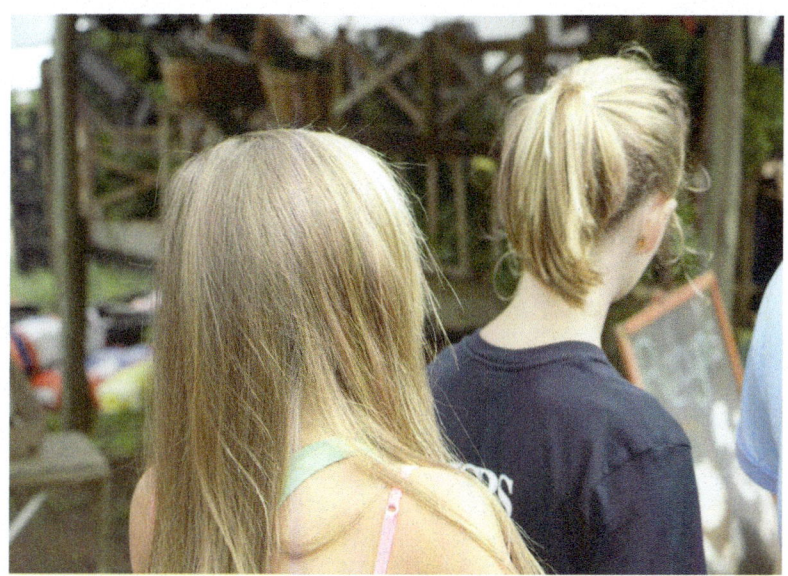

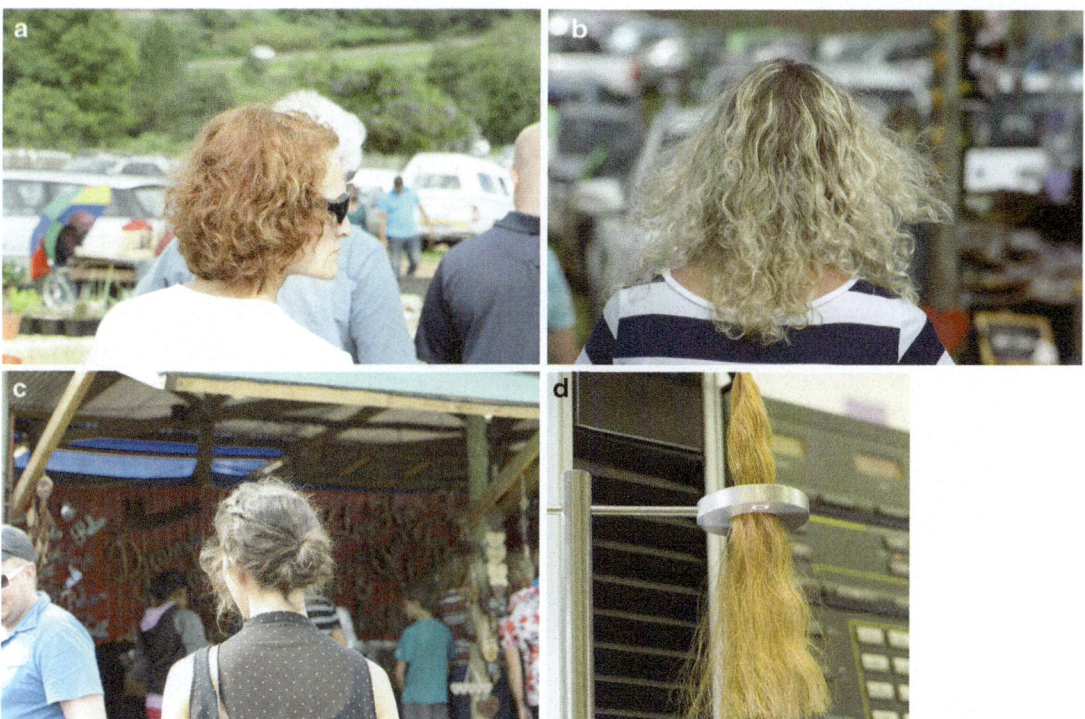

Fig. 2.25 (**a**, **b**, **c**) Manifestations of frizz; (**d**) frizz experimentally induced in the laboratory

sensitive to moisture and, in fact, was used in early hygrometer instruments to measure relative humidity. Women will often use a blow dryer or flat iron during styling to create their desired style. During drying, water is first removed from between fibers and then from inside each fiber. On removal, temporary hydrogen bonds form between protein chains, locking the alignment pattern in place. However, in high humidity water will diffuse back into hair and these bonds will be lost and replaced by water-protein hydrogen bonds. One consequence is return of hair to its

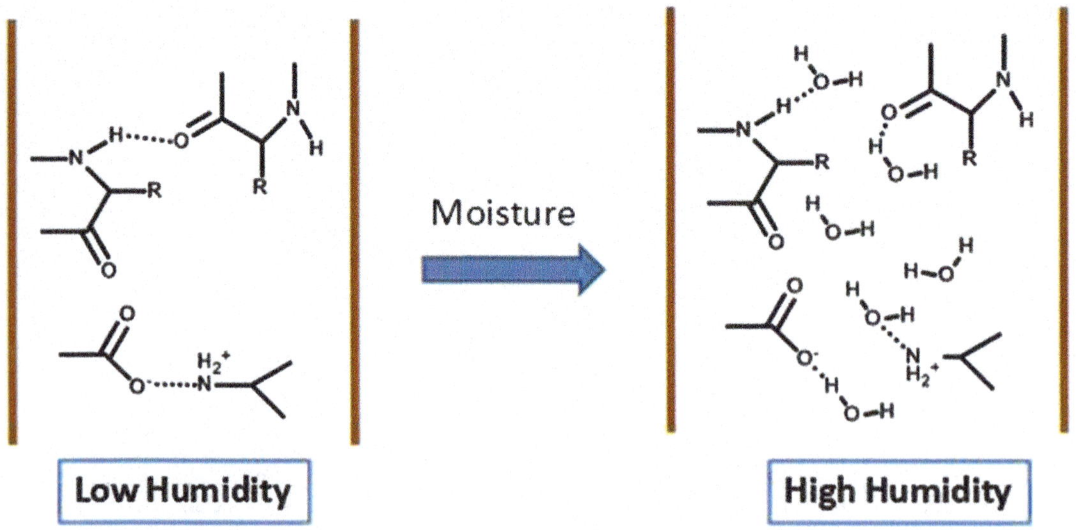

Fig. 2.26 Effects of low and high humidity

natural shape, and thus loss of created style. For women with straight hair who created curl, this can be seen as loss of volume and a flat look. For women with curly hair this can be seen as expansion or loss of alignment of curl (Fig. 2.26).

There is a tactile component of frizz which is driven in part by loss of alignment in high humidity and in part by surface changes. Hair without frizz feels softer, smoother, and significantly more moisturized.

Water diffusion into hair can be an enemy of style and smoothness, and makes any damage to hair more noticeable. However, many women believe that water is good for their hair and buy products to increase moisturization. This appears to be inconsistent, but it should be noted that moisturization is a consumer perception of conditioning properties, and not directly related to water content in hair. Damaged hair will feel dry due to surface changes and a rough texture. Broken fibers and split ends will also contribute to a dry feel perception by creating misalignment. Repairing this damage, e.g., via adding conditioning products or oils, is perceived as moisturization, but is in reality changing surface properties to make hair feel smoother.

Sign 4: Volume

Volume and, more importantly, the ability to achieve and keep volume, is a sign of hair health. This is especially true in regions of the USA and Europe where Caucasian hair types predominate. A commonly articulated requirement for volume is to frame the face in an attractive way. The other is lift at the roots, with a signal of unhealthy hair being hair that lies flat and limp against the scalp. However, it is often the signals of lack of volume that are key drivers of dissatisfaction. Hair that is thinning, stringy, greasy, limp, and clumped are all descriptors which indicate diminished volume (Fig. 2.27a, b).

Hair curvature, friction, stiffness, and fiber diameter will all increase volume, with fiber curvature playing the most important role. Caucasian hair is typically fine in diameter (60–80 μm vs. 80–100 μm for Asian hair). It is also much

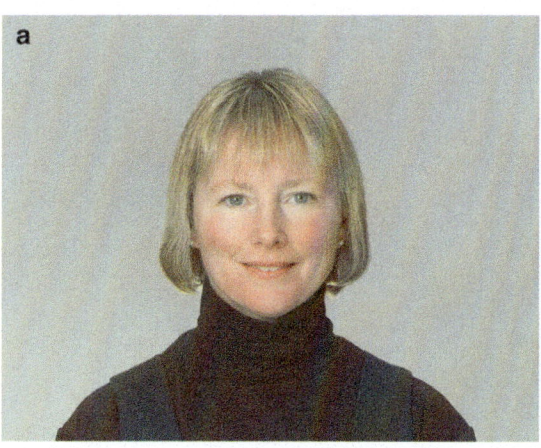 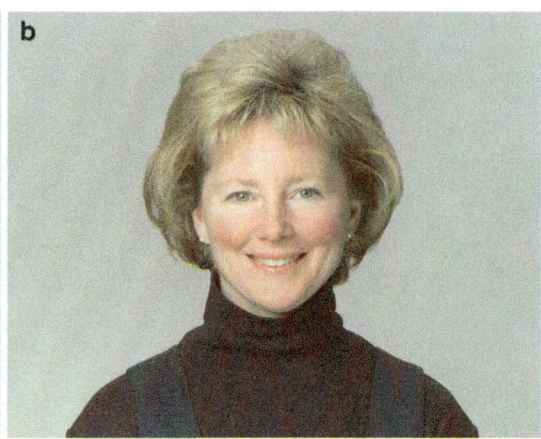

Fig. 2.27 Volume is a signal of hair health for some women, especially in regions such as the USA and Europe. Before (**a**) and after (**b**) the use of a volumizing regimen (see Chap. 6)

straighter than hair from women of either Asian or African descent. As a consequence, this hair type tends to lie flat against the face and have very little parting line volume. Straight hair will also increase the rate of sebum wicking, which will contribute to lack of volume several days after washing.

While this need for volume is more relevant in the US and European markets, it can still be relevant in East-Asian markets such as China and Japan where oily roots that require frequent washing and thin hair that is difficult to style are contributing to a woman's perception that her hair is not healthy.

These hair properties dictate some of the observed habits in these regions. Women looking to achieve volume will tend to have shorter hair styles in order to reduce the flat look. They also have a lower incidence of conditioner use and choose conditioners with lower silicone levels. To maximize root lift women will also only apply conditioner to hair tips vs. all over or use conditioners less frequently. These women often use more styling products to create stiffness and friction at the root.

Lack of volume as a signal of hair health becomes even more important as women age, and can be applicable to all women independent of hair type. As women age, hair gets finer in diameter and also less dense (i.e., fewer fibers per unit area of scalp). It is the combination of both of these effects that gives the appearance of loss of volume and typically is observed after the age of 45–50. In addition, especially with darker hair, the scalp skin maybe more visible as hair density decreases, which contributes to the perception of lack of volume and also hair health.

Sign 5: No Breakage/Strength

Hair is one of the strongest natural materials known. This property of hair is perceived as a highly important signal of hair health for all hair phenotypes. Advertising reinforces this perception by strongly linking hair strength with hair health via claims such as "3× stronger" after use of product. However, these claims are typically driven by conditioning actives that reduce surface friction, and thus breakage, vs. changing fundamental hair strength.

To many women a signal of weak hair is the appearance of fibers after brushing or in the shower drain. To note, some of this hair is almost certainly daily telogen loss (see Chap. 1) as a normal healthy scalp will lose approximately 50–100 fibers per day, but changes in this amount maybe noticed. Women may notice an increased number of shorter fibers, for example, in the area where a ponytail tie has been

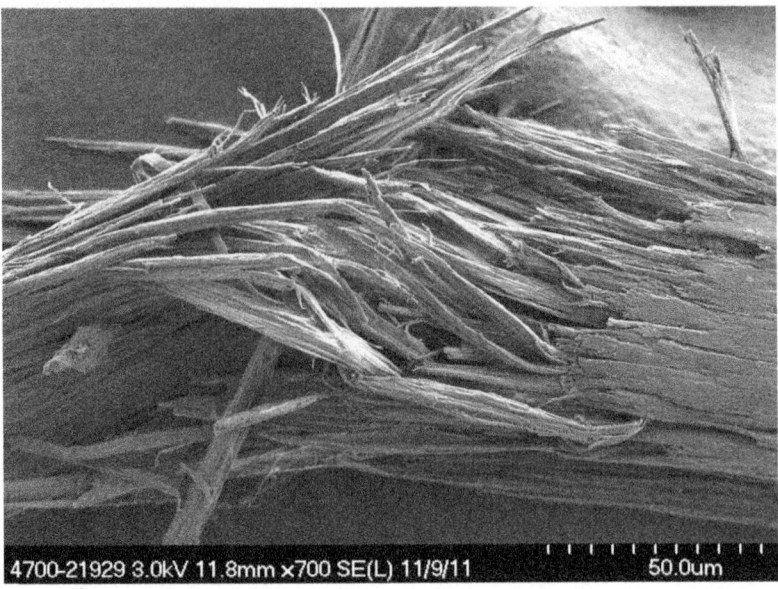

Fig. 2.28 Electron micrograph (EMG) image of broken hair fiber

used or where high heat has been frequently applied. As with damaged tips, the volume of a ponytail, frequency of needing haircuts, or inability to grow longer hair can also be signals of weaker hair. It is also recognized that "fine" hair is weaker than "coarse" hair. The lower diameter of fine hair can mean up to 140 % less protein. Consequently, women with fine hair will often describe their hair as weak.

It has been amply demonstrated that a single healthy hair will be pulled out of the scalp before it breaks by self pulling. However, as described, breakage can occur at tangles and knots as hair is brushed or combed. In addition, chemical treatments such as colorants and relaxers can weaken hair to make it more susceptible to this type of breakage. Often breakage in these circumstances can be observed in a light microscope or scanning electron microscope as an uneven break (Fig. 2.28).

Wet hair is easier to break than dry hair due to water being able to plasticize the protein structure by breaking the electrostatic interactions between protein chains. More breakage can occur when hair is wet, and additional care should be taken during wet combing. Conditioning products provide wet combing benefits to protect against this breakage.

In the next chapter, we examine the multiple causes of damage to the hair shaft, and the cumulative impact these have on hair health from root to tip.

References

1. Sinclair RD. Healthy hair: what is it? J Invest Derm Symp Proc. 2007;12(2):2–5.
2. Gray J, editor. International Congress & Symposium Series 266—assessment of hair quality using eye-tracking technology. London: RSM Press; 2006.

Understanding Hair Damage

Introduction: The Hair Mass

A single human hair grows at the rate of approximately 9–12 mm per month. The combined effect of approximately 100,000 hair shafts produces a physical entity—the hair mass—which increases at a combined total of approximately 6 feet (1.8 m) an hour or 140 feet (46.67 m) per day. At a uniform length of 40 cm, this represents 40 km of hair carried on the head. It is this mass which allows us to display hair in the manner of our choosing and is, in turn, dependent on the root-to-tip integrity of the 100,000 or so hair shafts on our scalp.

In this chapter, the different 'insults' to hair and how they change the hair's external and internal structure are examined.

Hair in Time and Space

It is important to recognise that hair exists in both time as well as space. During a glancing observation of a head of hair, the observer makes a subconscious assessment of hair as though it were all of the same chronological age. The reality is that for a head of hair, such as in Fig. 3.1, the temporal difference between roots and tips is almost 6 years. As an analogy, the gleaming car in the showroom would not look the same after 6 years on the road and being exposed to a myriad of insults and lack of care. The same applies to hair.

In theory, a day's growth of hair breaking the surface might remain in similar, if not identical, condition, until some years later; it is cut off or falls to the ground in the exogen phase. In children and young adults, preservation of good condition is possible. Adult female hair can survive relatively unscathed by a combination of good hair care and a sympathetic environment.

For most adults, there is both a natural and progressive deterioration in the internal and external condition of the hair shaft over time. This is the result of environmental and self-inflicted, repeated damage. This process known as **weathering** can vary from minimal to extreme (Fig. 3.2a, b).

In young women who do not use chemical processes or excessive heat on their hair, this weathering process is almost impossible to detect with the naked eye. In women with repeated chemical applications, the damage (Fig. 3.3a, b), particularly at the tip, is all too evident.

Modern research techniques now allow hair scientists and researchers to examine the breakdown of the structures of the hair at a nanoscale (i.e. the breakdown of chemical bonds). It is now possible to extrapolate not only how these breakdowns result in changes in a single fibre marker (such as loss of tensile strength) but also how these single fibre changes impact bulk properties such as noticeable shine. The extent of the structural changes and their manifestations will vary depending on the morphology of hair, i.e. diameter and curl and on the prevailing hair style (long vs. short).

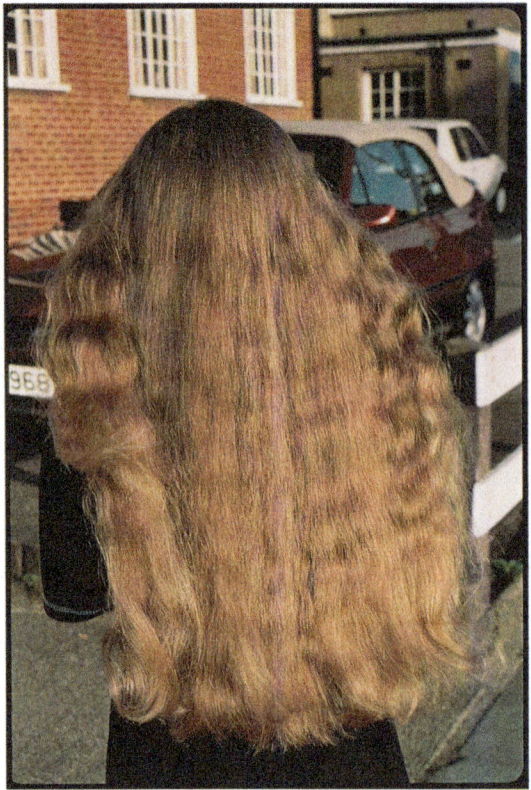

Fig. 3.1 Six years of uninterrupted growth and still showing signs of health

The Process of 'Weathering'

Hair is an exceptionally resilient structure able to withstand many differing traumas—environmental, mechanical, physical, and chemical. Hairs taken from ancient Egyptian mummies and even from the bodies of our Stone Age ancestors appear remarkably well preserved, even after thousands of years (Fig. 3.4).

In the twenty-first century, in spite of this resilience, badly weathered hair is epidemic, particularly in the developed world (Fig. 3.5a–d).

When hair first emerges from the scalp, the cuticle consists of up to 10 layers of long 'scales'. However, the cuticular layers are only 3 or 4 μm thick and may have to last for some 6 years or more.

Natural weathering involves a wearing away of the cuticle of the hair shaft, primarily from physical acts of grooming.

Accelerated weathering occurs as a result of additional and excessive physical and, most importantly, repeated chemical injury. This accelerated weathering, which is generally regarded as 'damage', involves destruction not only of the f-layer and damage to the cuticle but ultimate

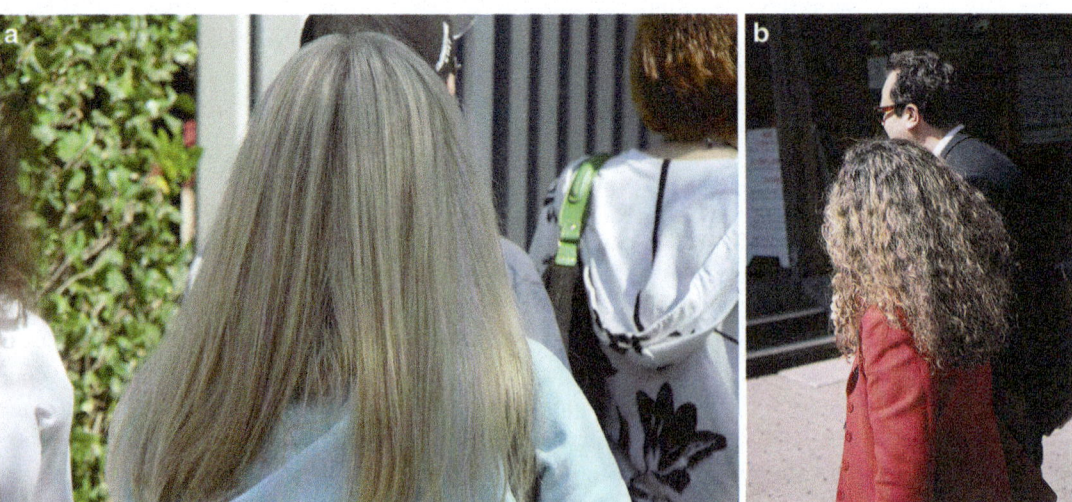

Fig. 3.2 (**a**) Minimal and (**b**) severe weathering

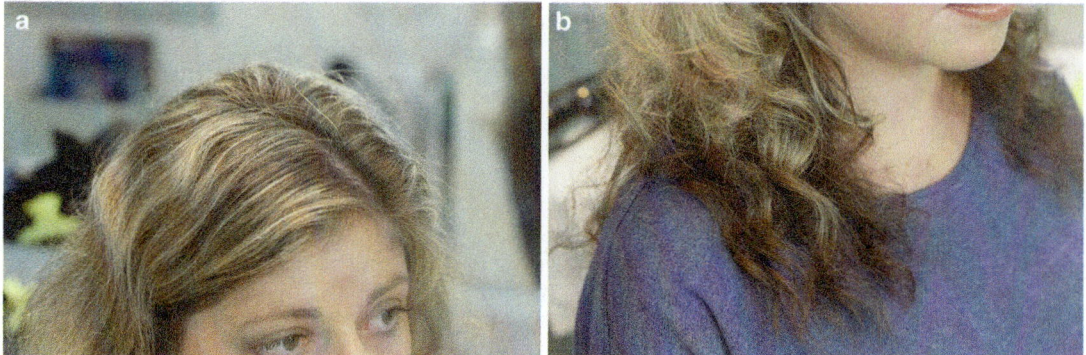

Fig. 3.3 The hair mass is some 40 km of hair. Note the difference in integrity from (**a**) root to (**b**) tip

Fig. 3.4 Henna-coloured hair which has survived thousands of years on an ancient Egyptian mummy. Courtesy of the Vatican Museum

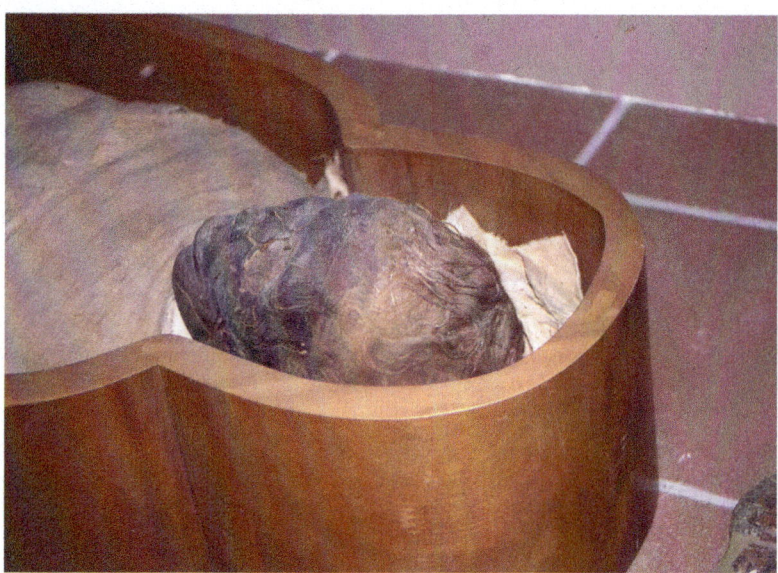

exposure and degradation of the proteins in the cortex. The latter becomes increasingly unable to maintain the structural and homeostatic integrity of the hair, and, at its most extreme, the hair proteins may unravel, causing split ends or breakage in mid-shaft (Fig. 3.6a–d).

Sources of Damage

Major damaging sources include wetting, friction, sunlight, heat from drying and styling appliances, and chemicals and heavy metals in swimming pools and even the home. Most devastating are chemical procedures, notably bleaching, perming, relaxing, and straightening.

Other insults are due to poor habits and practices and include the physical damage from brushing and combing and the use of excessive heat from implements such as blow dryers and flat irons. It is now recognised that poor brushing and combing are more detrimental than previously thought.

The Record of the Hair

Physical and chemical insults are permanently recorded along the length of a hair as it grows. Some can be seen with the naked eye, others only under the microscope. Such events may be regarded as the record of the hair (Fig. 3.7).

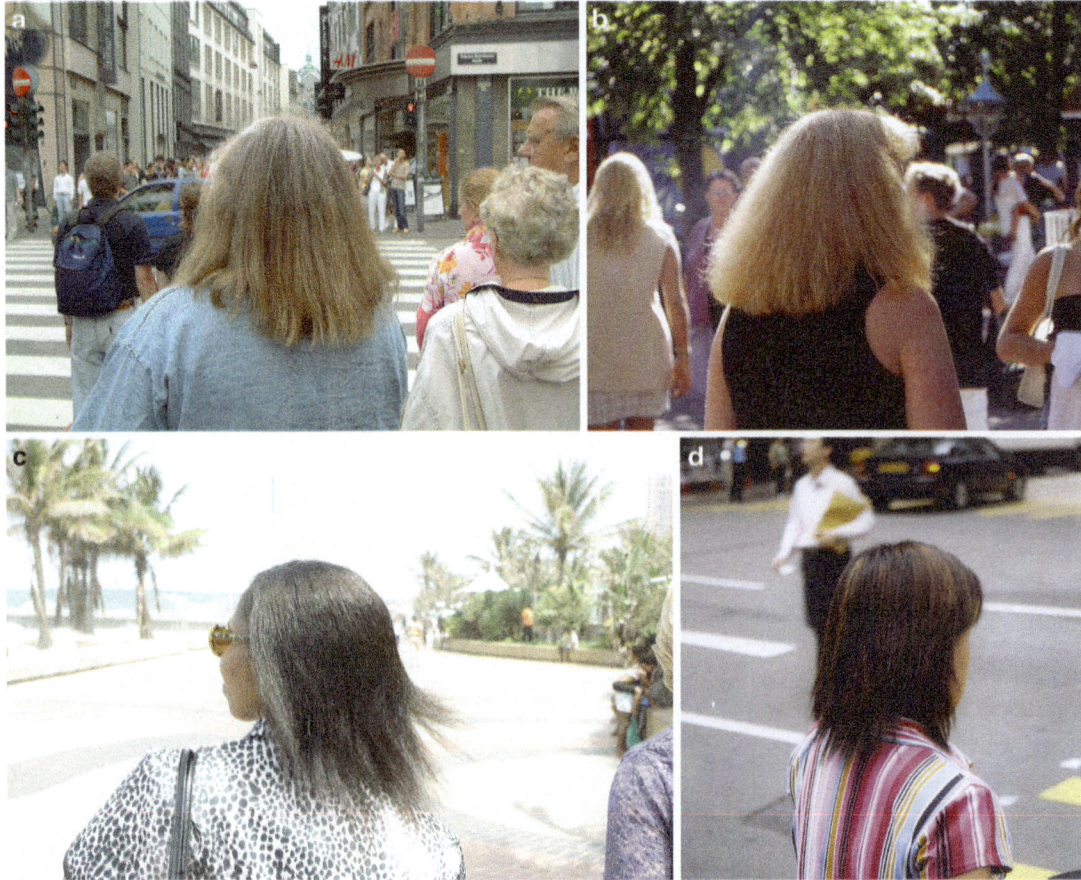

Fig. 3.5 In the twenty-first century, badly weathered hair is epidemic from (**a**) Copenhagen and (**b**) New York to (**c**) South Africa and (**d**) Singapore

Case Study
An extreme example of damage over time is exemplified by a Chinese woman who had an exceptionally long anagen phase and had not cut her hair for 26 years [1]. *She washed her hair twice a month, and the majority of time, the hair was kept wrapped in a turban, away from sun exposure. Some hair was longer than 4 m, but a full analysis was performed on intact hair that was 2–2.4 m long.*

A variety of analytical methods were used to investigate the hair samples, including assessing chemical changes (protein and lipids measurements), ultra structural changes (TEM, AFM EXPLAIN imaging), and physical parameters (shine, surface, diameter, and resistance measures). The lady had less damage than women who wash and use chemical treatments on their hair, but there was a clear degradation from root to tip of the hair structure. In particular, the damage appeared to manifest itself earliest in the cuticle region, followed by the cortical keratin-associated proteins (KAPs), and finally the cortical keratin network.

Causes of Hair Damage

Figure 3.8 shows an average exposure to these various insults over 1 year, which equates to approximately 12–15 cm of growth. The types of damage have been colour coded to four main processes—environmental, physical, heat, and chemical.

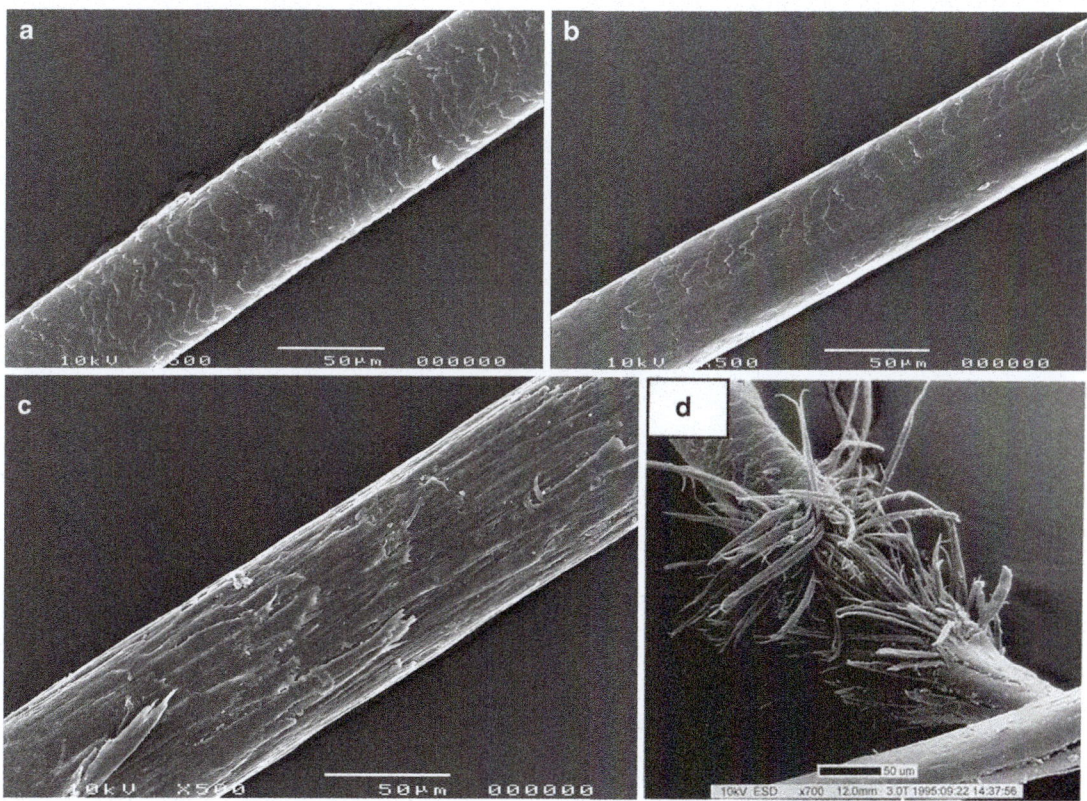

Fig. 3.6 Scanning Electron Microscope (SEM) images of progressive severe weathering to a hair shaft: (**a**) root, (**b**) mids, and (**c**) tips; (**d**) trichorrhexis nodosa, from a woman with 15 cm length hair

Fig. 3.7 The record of the hair

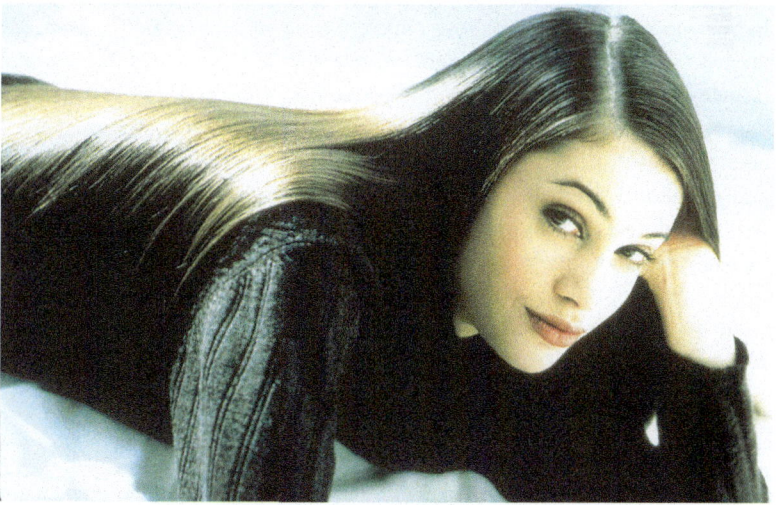

These insults do not occur in isolation. The final damage to hair is due to a combination of all these factors, their frequency, and intensity. If a woman possesses hair of 40 or 50 cm length, there may be 4 or 5 years of these cumulative insults on the hair ends.

Most of these insults impact the nano-structure of hair by causing changes to protein and lipid

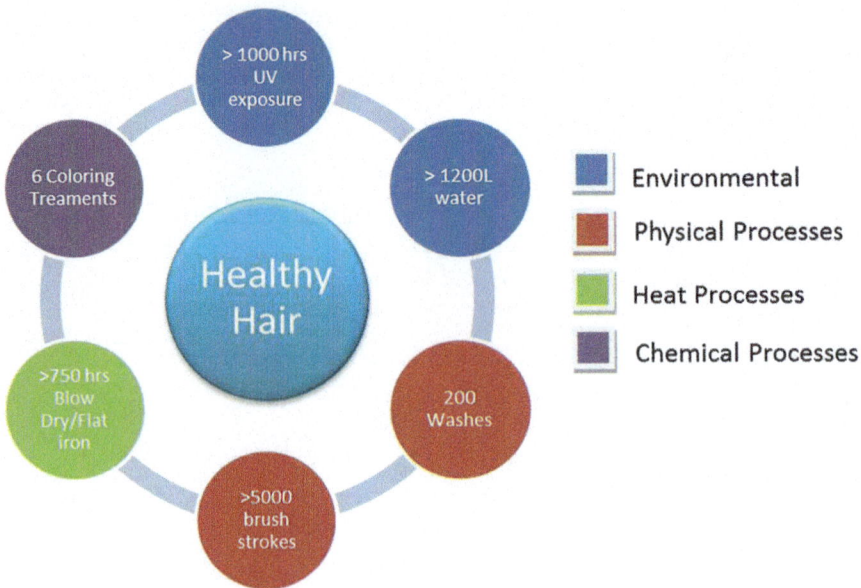

Fig. 3.8 Causes of hair damage

structures. The insults themselves cannot be detected, but can be measured by techniques such as proteomics and lipidomics that identify the exact structural changes (see Chap. 4).

As a result, there are microstructural and single fibre changes that eventually will manifest as macrostructural or bulk hair changes. As an increasing number of fibres lose cuticles, the cortex will eventually be exposed, which further reduces shine and will increase the propensity of hair to form split ends. As more protein damage occurs, the tensile strength of hair will decrease and eventually lead to breakage, which women will then notice as additional hairs in the brush or as a lack of smoothness from the broken ends.

Hair Damage: Women's Perspective

While the hair scientist, dermatologist, trichologist, and stylist all have a view on hair damage, it behoves all of them to determine whether women are both aware of the causes of hair damage and have any genuine concern. Without concern, compliance in the use of any treatment or haircare product is invariably destined for failure.

All too often, significant hair damage results in disappointment and an unhappy client, patient, or consumer. Repeated attempts to restore the hair to good condition, or create a requested style, may be doomed by a lack of understanding of the process.

Research shared in the previous chapter has indicated that hair damage is indeed of major and increasing concern to women. They manifestly see and feel signals that can be attributed to changes in hair structure resulting from damage. Most obvious are lack of shine, frizz, lack of strength (i.e. breakage), dry feel, and loss of volume. They also observe the changes toward the tips of their hair, most commonly light changes, split ends, and breakage (Fig. 3.9a–c).

Women's Perception of Causes of Damage

Women most frequently cite styling, especially regular use of heated implements (flat irons and blow dryers) as the major cause of hair damage. To a lesser extent, brushing and combing are believed to be implicated. Chemical treatments such as colouring and perming are also recognised

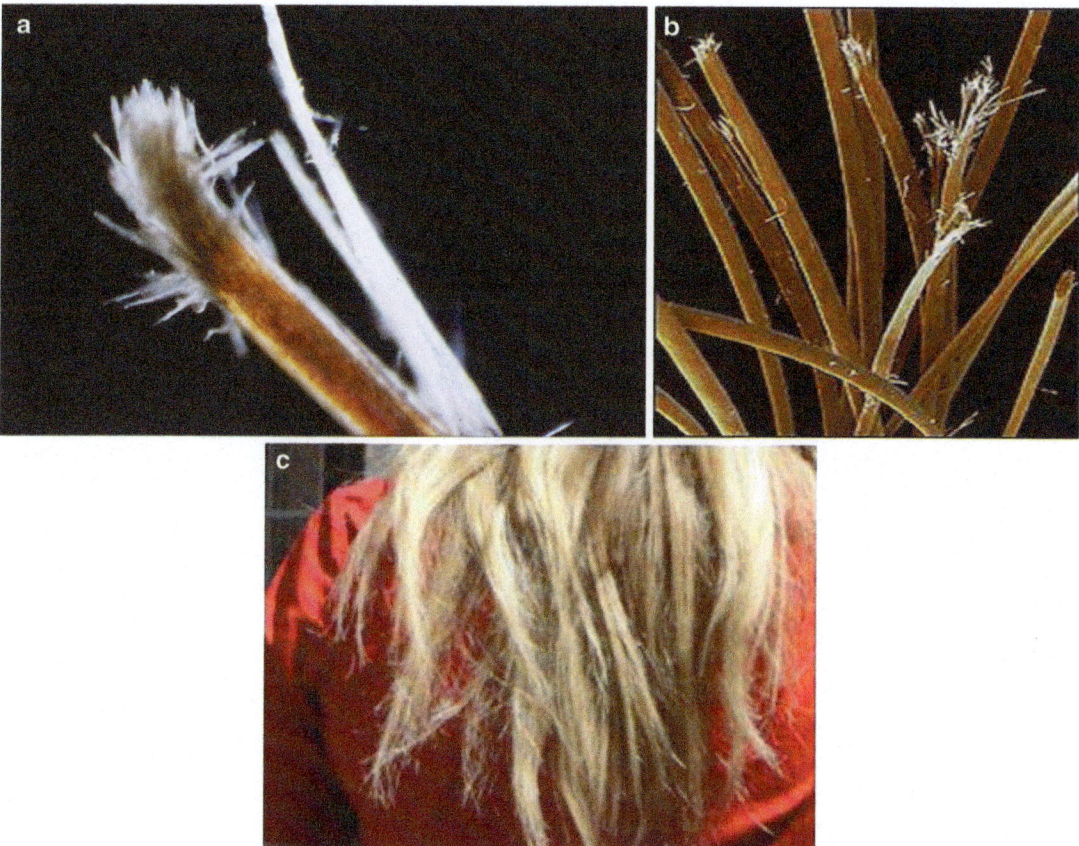

Fig. 3.9 (**a**) Split ends 3 cm from the scalp, (**b**) under the microscope, to (**c**) the awful reality

to be damaging. A majority of women continue to colour, but not as often as they wish, recognising the impact of these procedures.

To a portion of the population, more overtly damaging treatments such as bleaching or relaxing are undertaken as infrequently as possible to avoid overprocessing. Women using these treatments will often change their styling habits to minimise further damage, using, for example, a lower heat setting on the blow dryer or using a wide-toothed comb to avoid tangles.

Global Perspective

Around the world, the same categories are seen as damaging, i.e. chemical treatments, heat styling, and physical damage (brushing and combing), but there are differences in the degree of importance depending on habits and practices in different regions.

Hair colouring is more popular for women with Indo-European phenotype hair in the USA and consequently rated higher as a significant cause of damage. Women in Japan and Mexico also rate hair colouring as being highly damaging. Similarly, chemical relaxing is more common among women of African descent and is a significant cause of hair damage for this group.

Curly/flat iron usage is lower in Asian countries such as China and Japan, and thus, not surprisingly, these implements are rated lower for causing damage than in countries such as the USA, UK, and Mexico.

Interestingly, getting older/more mature is a cause of lower hair health for 20–25 % of the population, especially for women past the age of 35 years. It is higher in Japan, around 40 %, and this may be due to a higher focus on ageing in the beauty products area in this country.

Summary

Women expressing concern about their lack of healthy hair do recognise that it is essentially their actions which are causing this damage, and there is an associated element of guilt. Styling and colouring are known to be damaging, but are felt to be necessary to achieve the look women are seeking. A constant struggle exists to balance final look with a desire to have healthy hair. Women believe that if hair is unhealthy, it will be more difficult to achieve the desired style, so it is even more important to keep hair healthy.

Psychological Consequences of Unhealthy Hair

Perception of healthy hair is not only a desire to look beautiful, but it is also linked to how confident an individual feels and how others perceive them. Research scientists have attempted to quantify the causes other than mere visible damage behind the notorious 'bad hair day'.

Bad Hair Day Study

Much anecdotal evidence supports the contention that a bad hair day is associated with the mood of the individual. In an attempt to correlate the physical manifestations of bad hair, a study at the University of Sheffield followed women over a 3-month period with the intent of assessing whether there was a scientific explanation of a 'bad hair day' [1]. Assessments included subjects maintaining a diary of their hair-care habits and practices and recording their menstrual cycles. Subjects also maintained a record of positive or negative feelings throughout the 3-month study. Objective observations of hair quality, including styling, were made by the investigators, and measurements of daily scalp sebum were taken.

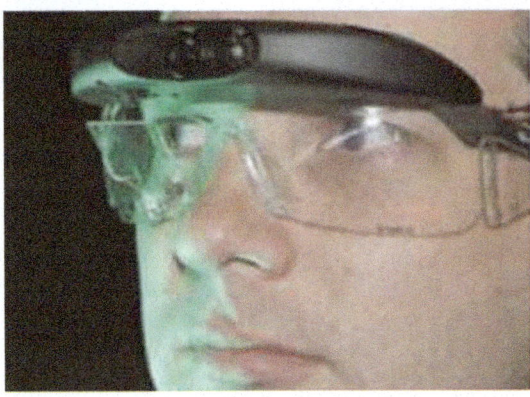

Fig. 3.10 Eye-tracker technology uses a camera- or video-based system to accurately monitor the movements of the eye

Among many interesting data, the study revealed that a 'bad hair day' seemed to coincide with the onset of menstruation and was intimately related to a decrease in hair washing and conditioning and a sharp reduction in grooming and styling. Conversely, the 'best hair day' coincided with ovulation. No evidence for greasy hair being associated with sebum levels was found.

This study suggests that grooming habits may be associated with the normal menstrual cycle and are a reflection of hair as a sexual signal.

Hair and Face as Social Signals

Social anthropologists have suggested that although the hair is a key human signal, particularly at a distance, it is the face to which humans are most attracted at close quarters. However, when hair is dishevelled, dirty, or otherwise unharmonious, it is thought to distract the eye and to diminish the overall appearance of beauty and health. Studies to investigate this have employed a novel device—eye-tracker technology

Eye-Tracker Technology

Other aspects of the social effects of unhealthy hair are highlighted by research conducted in the USA and France utilising eye-tracker technology. An eye tracker is a novel device used to discretely measure and record eye positions and eye movements (Fig. 3.10). Although it has now been

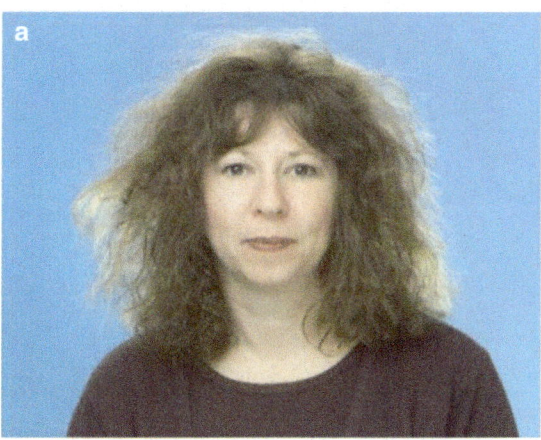 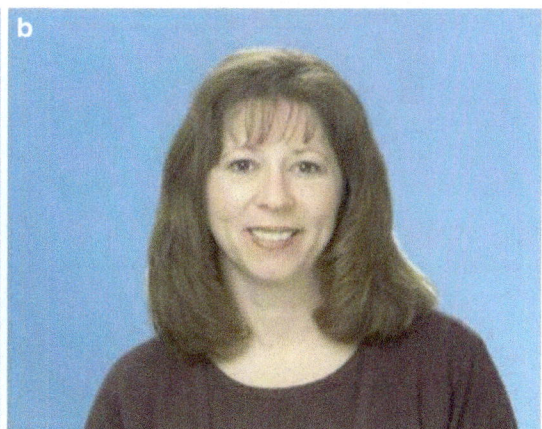

Fig. 3.11 A clinical study using eye-tracker technology investigated the hypothesis that (**a**) dry, damaged, and unhealthy hair distorts the observers' perception of (**b**) attractiveness

applied as a research tool for a variety of human tasks, it was developed originally to assess the eye movements of fighter pilots when controlling fast jets.

Eye trackers are used in research into the visual system, in psychological evaluation, and in product design. The most common purpose of eye tracking is to estimate change of direction of gaze in order to determine precisely what a person is most frequently looking at. This latter is referred to as the 'gaze plot'. Eye-tracking technology uses a camera- or video-based system to accurately monitor the movements of the eyes; a computer displays the gaze frequency and plot, superimposed on the photos of the study subject.

Eye movements can be assessed while one person is subconsciously or deliberately 'inspecting' another. This approach lends itself more to examination of photographs than 'live' observations, where the obfuscating factors of embarrassment and reactionary bias may occur.

A clinical study was conducted to investigate the hypothesis that dry, damaged, and unhealthy hair distorts the observers' perception of attractiveness. Utilising eye-tracker technology, the eye movements and gaze plots of observers viewing photographic images of women whose hair displayed different characteristics were recorded. In addition, the study explored the hypothesis that healthy (shiny) hair enhances observers' perceptions of attractiveness (Figs. 3.11a, b, and 3.12).

The conclusions from the study suggested that:

- If hair is damaged, the eye lingers on this area for an increased time.
- The time taken to focus on hair in poor condition results in less time being taken to observe the face, which detracts from facial features (attractiveness).
- If hair is in good condition (shiny/'healthy'), hair gaze time tends to be short.
- Panellists were asked whether the face or hair was more important in the beauty rating and which type of hair (good or bad) was more noticeable. Although several chose the face as most important, most commented that beauty is a combination of face and hair.
- Panellists noted that hair enhances the attractiveness rating when it complements the face and can detract if the hairstyle is distracting (e.g. if it is 'flyaway', 'frizzy', or too long, or has poor fit with face shape). Results with female panellists were similar to those with male panellists.
- When hair had been styled, more time was spent on facial features. Other distractions were centre partings and widow's peaks.

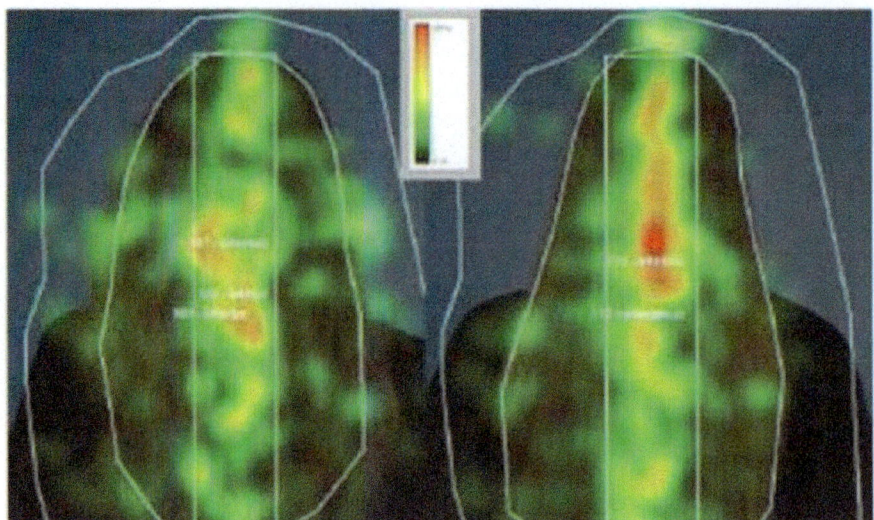

Fig. 3.12 Ungroomed left, groomed right. Gaze plot from eye-tracker technology. The more groomed the hair, the greater the observer's perception of healthy hair

- Women tended to give higher attractiveness ratings than men and were more likely than men to assume the model was younger when seen with 'good' hair from the back.
- A high rating of attractiveness was attributed to healthy, shiny hair and uniform curls, which were cited as sexually attractive. Eye-tracker data supported this conclusion, with higher resting times on areas of shine and well-defined curls.

When asked to explain why a high rating of attractiveness was given to these pictures, panellists used the following words/phrases: 'curls [are] uniform', 'hair looks healthy and shiny', '[I wonder] what product she uses', 'looks more professional', 'women look sexy with curly hair', 'looks shiny', 'silky, smooth', 'healthy', 'not dry', '[model is] someone who cares about her looks', and 'someone who spent time on her hair'.

In a similar study by Bernard Fink in 2013, test subjects viewed a series of healthy and damaged hair images and ranked them for age, health, and attractiveness. In all cases, there were significantly higher scores for undamaged/healthy hair [2].

From these studies, it is evident that hair is a critical factor in how people judge each other and assess physical attractiveness. Hair in good condition has a positive overall effect on the perception of that person, and shiny hair is a critical factor in how people judge 'beauty'.

Experimental Evidence of Root-to-Tip Hair Damage

Research scientists are now able to identify and quantify the damage which occurs to the hair shaft. The scanning electron microscope (SEM) is an invaluable research and teaching tool, allowing detailed examination of damage to the cuticle and, in severe cases, the cortex.

The graph below (Fig. 3.13) shows cuticle integrity for hair from 10 individuals with ~30 cm long hair, where the cuticle was assessed at the roots, mid-section, and tips using an SEM. Fifty fibres were graded on a 0–5 scale depending on the level of cuticle damage observed, and then the final grade calculated as shown below, where the maximum possible score is 250. In addition, representative images are shown illustrating the cuticle degradation (Fig. 3.14).

The data above shows microstructural changes to cuticle integrity that is easily measurable using SEM techniques and correlates well with the level of damage noticed by women.

Experimental Evidence of Root-to-Tip Hair Damage

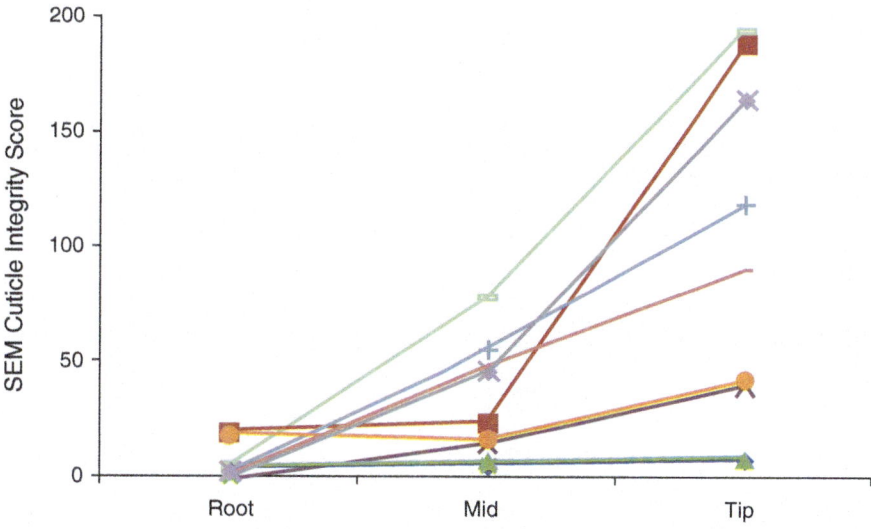

Fig. 3.13 SEM Score = (0*none) + (1*low) + (3*medium) + (5*stripped). Maximum score = 250

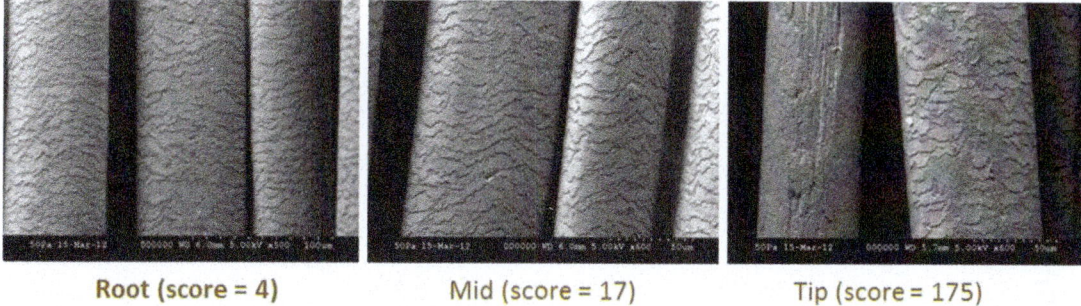

Fig. 3.14 Hair cuticle degradation, scored with SEM

Nano-structural changes are also measured root to tip from individual ponytails and specifically the degradation of proteins. These changes are not directly observable but will lead to a weakening of hair, making it more susceptible to further breakage. One manifestation of this protein degradation will be loss of tensile strength (i.e. how easy the fibre is broken).

The data below (Fig. 3.15) is from a set of 26 individual ponytails of ~30 cm long, where the protein degradation was measured by protein loss. This measure involves shaking a small sample of hair in water for an hour and the total amount of protein eluted into solution quantified using the Lowry method. The data below is for break load averaged across all the root ends vs. tip ends. Significant differences are observed between root values and tip values.

Damage Insults

It is possible to categorise the damage insults into four separate areas, which all contribute to root-to-tip strand health. These four categories are summarised in Fig. 3.16.

The relative importance of these categories will *vary from person to* person depending on their habits, their hair morphology and, to some extent, on their lifestyle and global location.

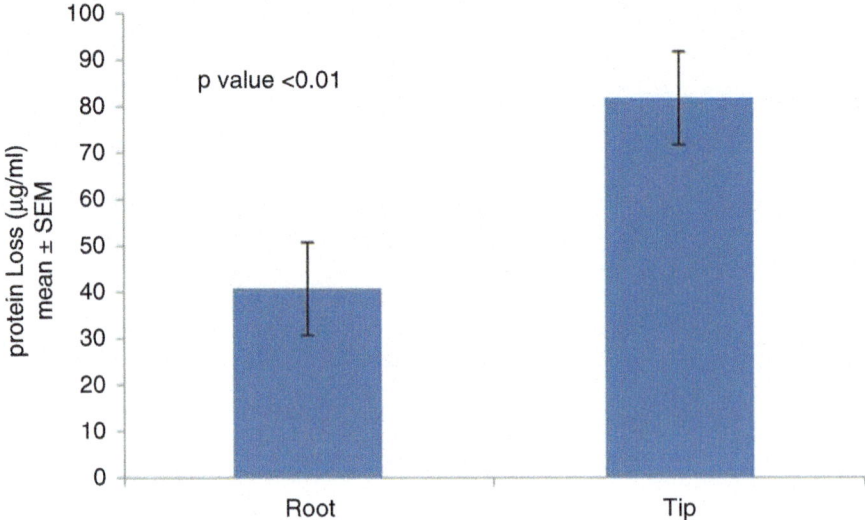

Fig. 3.15 Break load averaged across root ends vs. tip ends

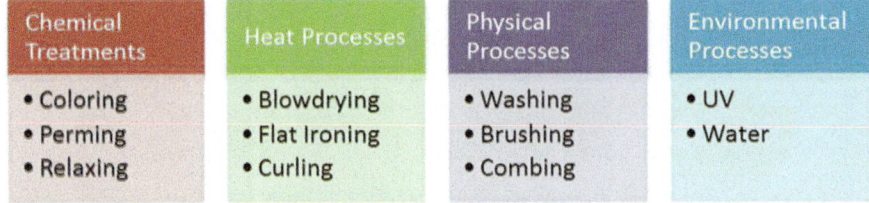

Fig. 3.16 Four separate areas which all contribute to root-to-tip strand health

It is not possible to assign a definitive figure on the percent contribution of each of these four areas to overall damage. However, it is possible to create a general hierarchy: chemical treatments that are the most damaging, followed by high and extended heat processes, followed by vigorous combing/brushing without products containing conditioning actives. Environmental processes tend to be lower in overall damage.

The extent of damage to hair and manifestation of this damage will depend on frequency and severity of these insults and on the resilience of hair. Figure 3.17 demonstrates this continuum of nano- to micro- to macro-changes that ultimately leads to observable hair damage (Figs. 3.18 and 3.19).

Specific Forms of Damage

In this section, the specific causes of damage to the hair are discussed: damage from hair cutting, styling, and shampooing.

Cutting

Cutting hair with blunt scissors results in a cut with a long, jagged edge; the cuticle scales are especially vulnerable to further damage. Stylists use high-quality steel scissors, which are very sharp and cut cleanly. It is possible to tell whether a stylist chose to use scissors or a razor by looking at the record of the hair: razor cutting produces long, tapering sections of cuticle which weather quickly and even peel back (Fig. 3.20).

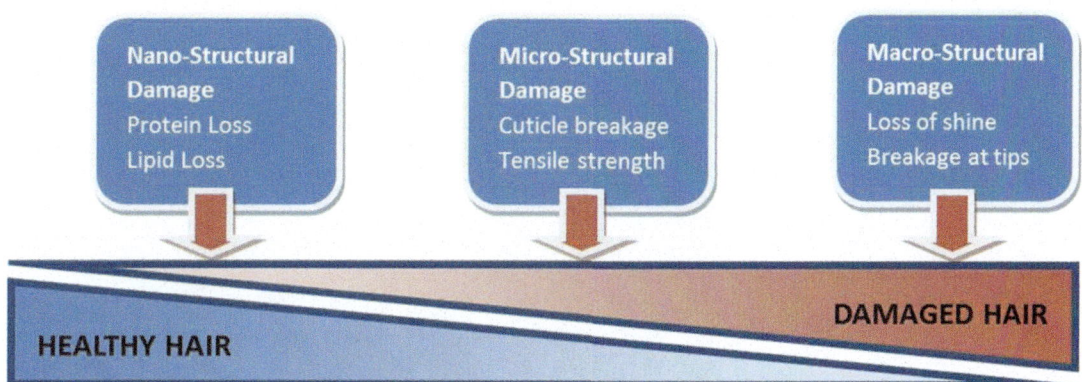

Fig. 3.17 Continuum of nano- to micro- to macro-changes that ultimately lead to observable hair damage

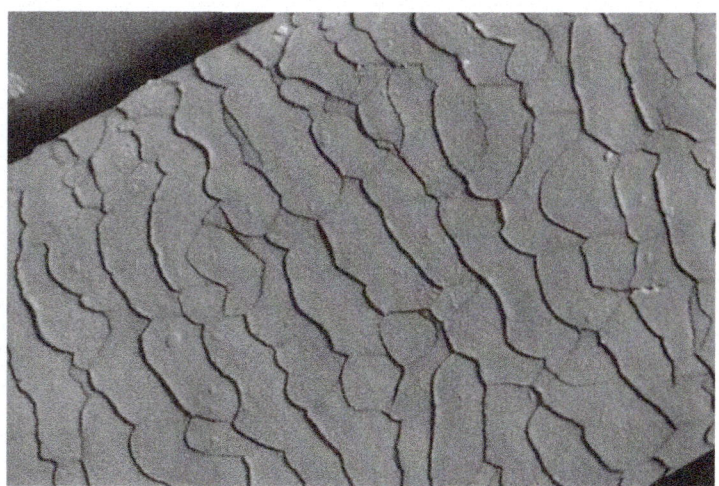

Fig. 3.18 Scanning Electron Microscope image of normal hair

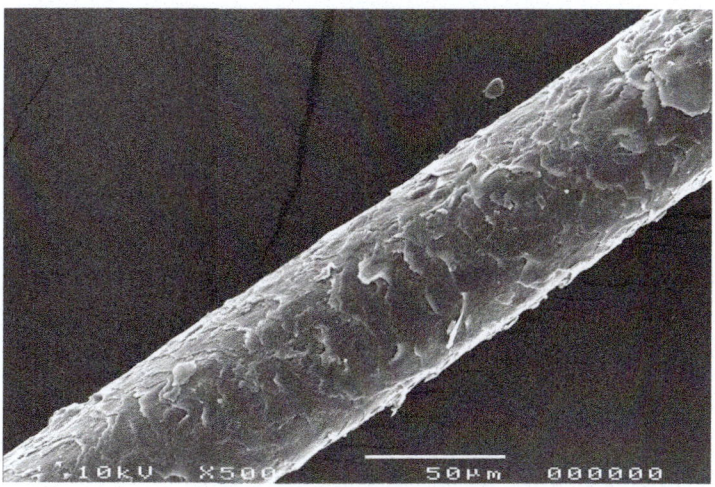

Fig. 3.19 Scanning Electron Microscope image of damaged hair; note the cuticle has cracked and split away

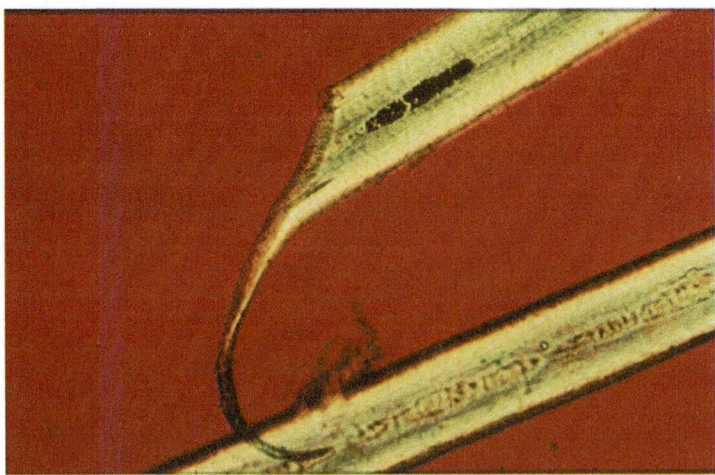

Fig. 3.20 Razored hair with incomplete cut leads to potential for peel back

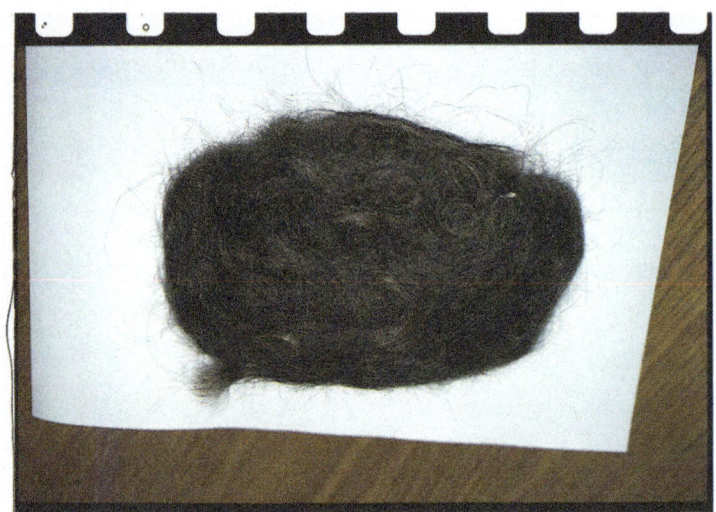

Fig. 3.21 Bird's nest hair—a form of felting due to physical interlocking of processed hair

Cutting hair when dry, in the belief that this will save the hair from heavy brushing when it is damp and therefore vulnerable to damage, is erroneous.

Styling

Plastic wide-toothed combs are less physically damaging to the hair than narrow, particularly metal, combs. Metal implements are also more prone to induce a static charge to hair and increase flyaway and frizz. A circular or semi-circular brush is probably the least damaging to hair.

Shampooing

In the past, when harsh shampoos were used, acute and even irreversible tangling or matting was often observed. Modern high-quality shampoos contain low levels of conditioning agents (see Chap. 5), which reduce this problem.

Tangling

Tangling of hair during shampooing may occur, particularly if the hair is long. At its worst, this can result in the so-called bird's nest hair, which is a form of felting, invariably associated with highly processed hair which interlocks (Fig. 3.21). It is often and falsely blamed on shampoo products when in fact it is a pure physical process. The only option in this instance is to cut the hair off.

Fortunately, this kind of matting is seldom seen nowadays, since most modern shampoos

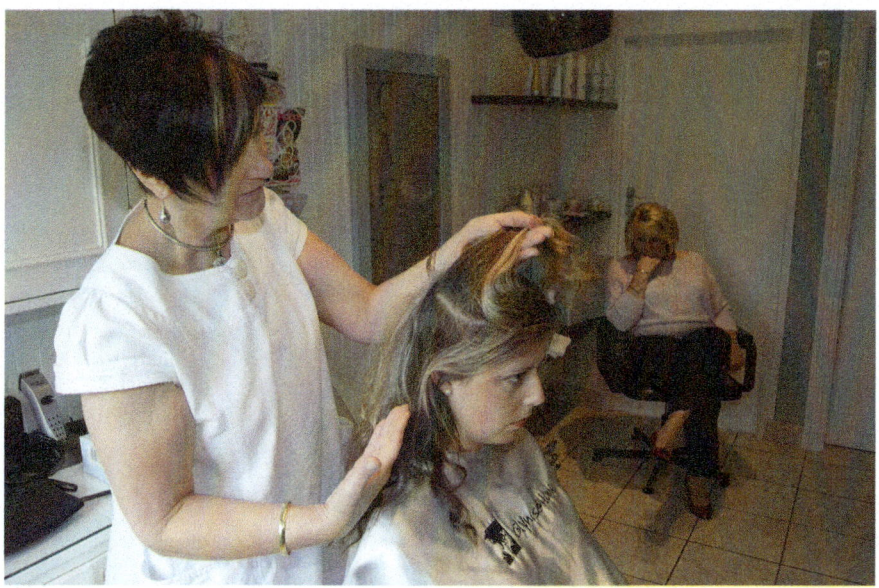

Fig. 3.22 Professional stylist showing that segmentation of hair before shampooing avoids tangling

contain conditioning agents designed to specifically reduce tangling. However, small amounts of tangling and, occasionally, matting are still quite common in long and weathered hair. It may be the result of wetting and drying hair without shampoo, since friction is higher in wet hair than in dry. It is sensible to segment long hair before shampooing to reduce this risk (Fig. 3.22).

Physical Processes

Hair is a highly resilient structure and has been designed to withstand what can amount to a huge number of physical processes over its lifetime. The cuticle, with multiple layers, imparts significant resistance, and the f-layer helps to decrease surface frictional forces. The cuticle has great internal strength, with a surface that has low friction, and if a cuticle cell is removed, the cuticle cell below is merely left exposed with a fresh surface.

A woman may brush her hair up to 1000 strokes per month with the consequence that the cuticle structure is degraded and eventually all the cuticles may be removed to reveal the less resilient cortex structure. The degradation due to these physical processes can take several forms. The first is abrasion of the cuticle edges, eventually leading to complete removal. Combing and brushing wet hair is more likely to lead to cuticle abrasion than combing and brushing dry hair, due to higher friction forces (Fig. 3.23).

Breakage may occur during combing and brushing. Under normal circumstances, the force required to pull a hair fibre out of the follicle is less than the force required to break a hair fibre. It might therefore be predicted that broken fibres would be rare. However, several factors can lead to broken fibres occurring. Excess chemical, UV, and heat exposure can eventually weaken hair sufficiently to lower the force to break hair below that required to pull hair out of the scalp. If the fibre is caught up in a knot during combing, the local forces in the knot can be much higher, causing the fibre to break. Breakage is especially an issue for curly hair since it is more likely to form tangles and knots leading to breakage, especially when wet.

Physical processes causing cuticle damage and breakage will occur for almost all women, but the severity of damage will vary according

Fig. 3.23 Cuticular peel back due to excessive grooming force

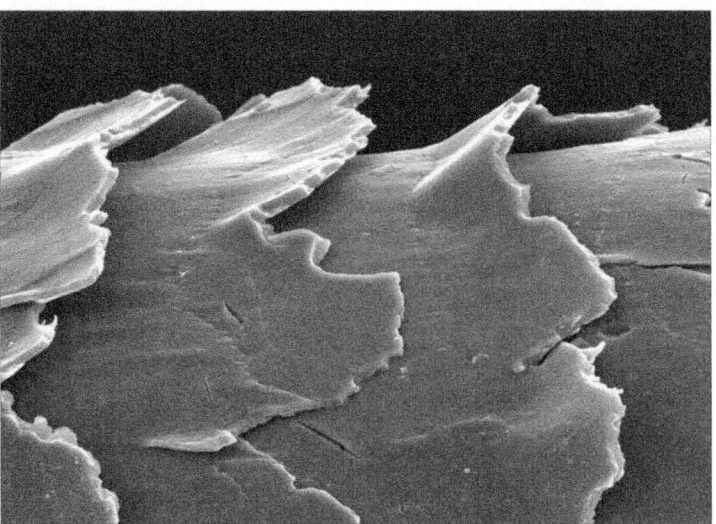

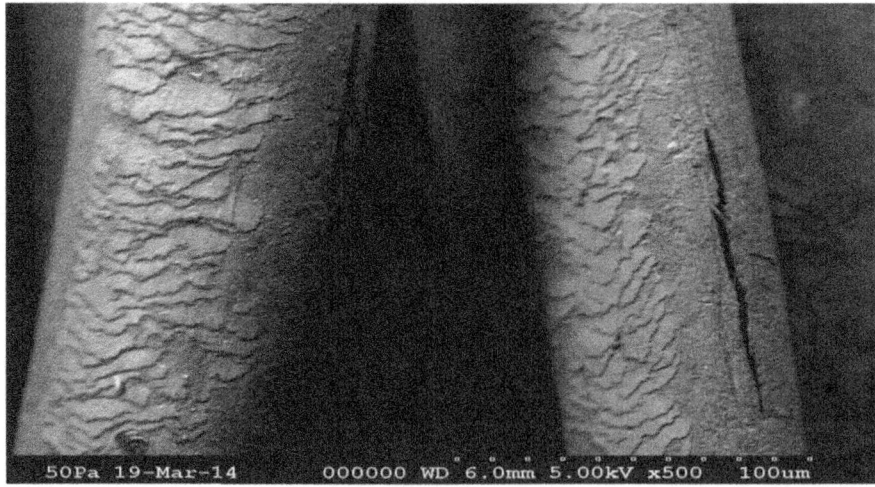

Fig. 3.24 SEM image of African American hair showing preferential abrasion at outside of hair

to hair morphology and habits and practices. Fine hair is more likely to break than thick hair simply because it has a lower tensile strength. Curly hair is more likely to break than straight hair due to higher abrasive forces between fibres and the likelihood of forming knots and tangles (Figs. 3.24 and 3.25). This is especially the case for women of African descent whose hair can be extremely fragile, especially if it has been regularly braided. Often, cuticle removal is seen preferentially on the outside edges of the fibre, as this is the part of hair where frictional forces are highest. Products that include conditioning actives such as quats and silicones are hugely impactful in helping to reduce this physical damage and work by creating lower frictional forces on the hair surface, thus making combing easier, with lower knot and tangle formation (see Chap. 5).

Environmental Processes

The hair of all women is exposed to the 'environment'. Unless they cover their hair for cultural or religious reasons, there will be some impact from the sun. UV exposure and its impact on hair have been widely studied. There are changes to the underlying hair structure by breaking down the protein structure, but also more visible signs after high levels of UV exposure. Extended exposure to sunlight can bleach melanin, giving hair a highlighted look, especially in lighter shades where melanin levels are lower and the bleaching effect is more obvious, i.e. medium blonde and lighter (Fig. 3.26a, b). Women with medium brown hair and darker may never observe melanin bleaching. Women may also notice permanent hair dyes being bleached by UV, but this may be less easy to distinguish vs. washing processes that can also rapidly fade dyes.

Hair is exposed to light, which is made up of a combination of different wavelengths, from UV to visible to infrared light (Fig. 3.27). The atmosphere and ozone layer will filter out some of UVC light, and window glass will filter out UVB, so lifestyle and time spent outdoors will influence the level of light exposure. In addition, the irradiance (i.e. the radiant power per unit area) will vary according to time of year and location. As an example, irradiance in summer sun is ~0.55 W/m^2 compared to 0.35 W/m^2 in winter sun.

The mechanisms of UV damage are complex, but it has been well established that all the components of hair structure are affected, including proteins, lipids, and melanin.

In the protein structure, the major amino acid residues that are impacted are the sulphur-containing residues cystine and methionine and the aromatic-containing residues tryptophan, tyrosine, and phenylalanine. The aromatic amino acids strongly absorb in the UV, forming excited state species which eventually form reactive oxygen species such as singlet oxygen, hydrogen peroxide, and hydroperoxides. The scheme

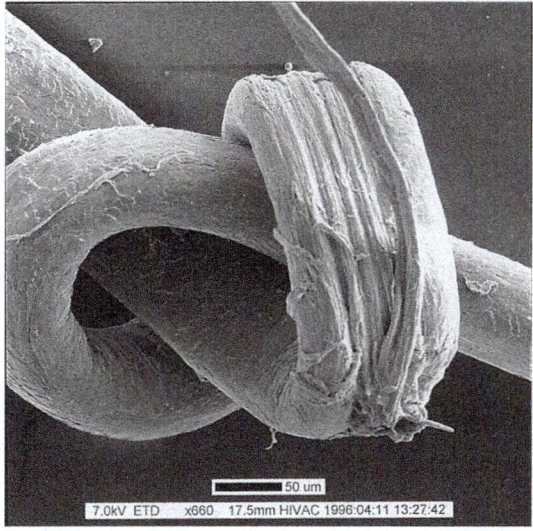

Fig. 3.25 Scanning Electron Microscope image of knots in hair

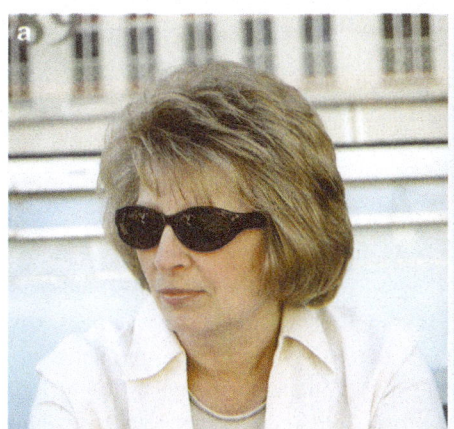
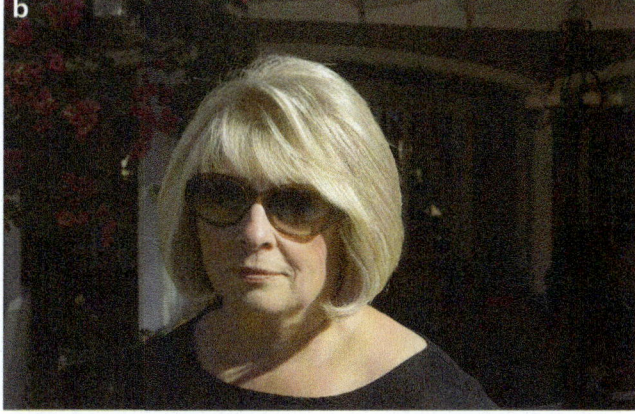

Fig. 3.26 Natural blonde (**a**) living in Europe and (**b**) after 4 years living in South Africa. Extended exposure to sunlight can bleach melanin, giving hair a highlighted look, especially in lighter shades where melanin levels are lower and the bleaching effect is more obvious

Fig. 3.27 Solar energy distribution

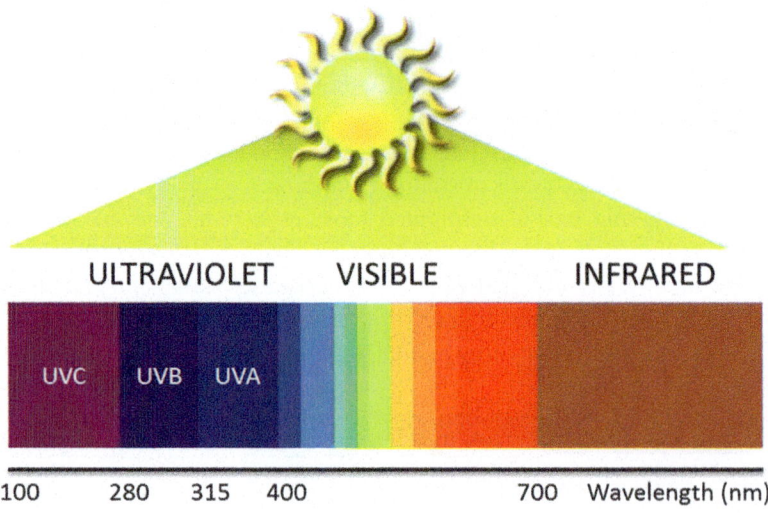

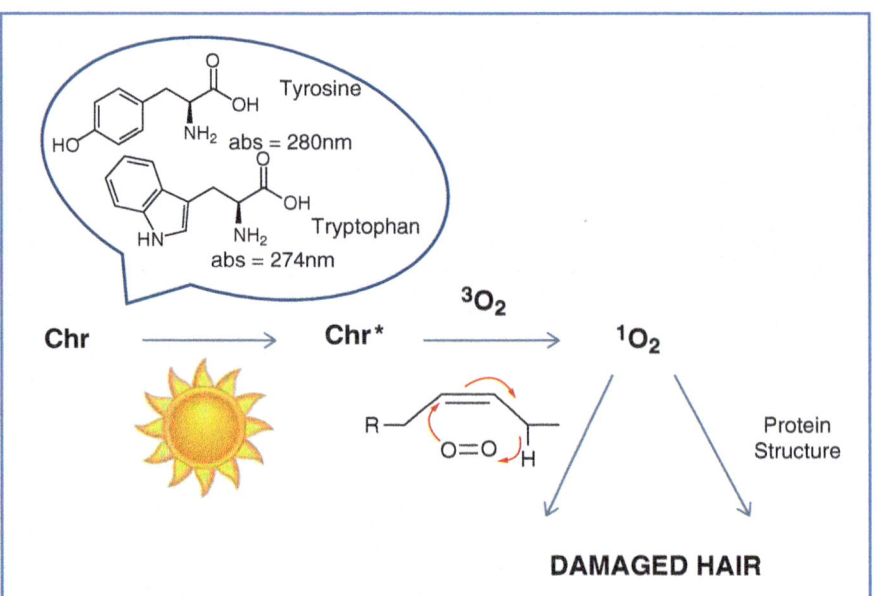

Fig. 3.28 Pathway to damaged hair from UV exposure

below shows basic pathways that can occur where proteins and lipids are slowly broken down via reaction with formed reactive oxygen species, in this case singlet oxygen (Fig. 3.28). Contaminants in hair such as copper ions have been shown to accelerate these damage mechanisms by creating additional reactive oxygen species [3]. Several oxidation products in the protein structure have been identified, including kynurenines, which are yellow in colour and are thought to be responsible for a photoyellowing of hair that is sometimes observed in grey hair.

Since all the hair structural components are susceptible to UV damage, many different hair properties are impacted. These include hair strength, both dry and wet, and also increased combing forces. Thus, hair exposed to UV may look lighter at the tips, but it may also look less

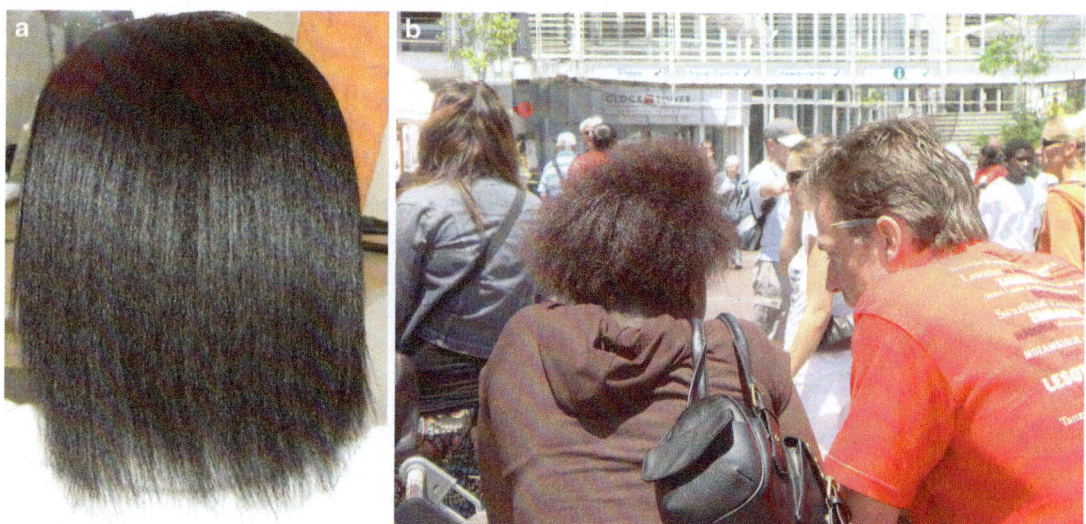

Fig. 3.29 Heat straightening is popular in Africa, with (**a**) good and (**b**) bad results

healthy, as structural damage manifests itself as broken fibres and split ends. All hair types will be impacted by UV damage although it is documented that darker hair will experience less damage due to the protective effect of melanin, which will also strongly absorb light. In addition, it is documented that artificial dyes will offer a protective effect by acting as UV absorbers [4] and it is also known that these dyes are oxidised and destroyed during this process.

Water is an important part of the hair-care process and can have beneficial effects by removing sebum lipids and dirt/dust from hair during the washing process. In some cases, it can also contain harmful metals, such as copper and iron, which are absorbed by hair. As mentioned elsewhere in this chapter, it has been demonstrated that copper absorbed by hair can accelerate damage from oxidative process such as hair colouring and UV exposure [5]. Water hardness, i.e. calcium and magnesium ions, can also impact hair health and also impact product performance. For example, in hard water, deposition of conditioning actives such as silicones is reduced, and lather amount is also reduced.

Heat Processes

There are a range of different structural changes caused by heat, but the factors crucial to determine the extent of these changes are firstly the temperature that the hair gets to and, secondly, the cumulative time of exposure to this temperature. Many women can use heat implements without noticeable damage if they take care with frequency of use and moderate the temperature of the device. However, the benefits women are looking for with heat implements, e.g. curl formation or straightening, are correlated with the level of heat used, so it can often be a trade-off between level of damage and desired style achievement. For some women, heat implements are used simply to dry hair, but the majority are using heat implements as a tool to style hair.

Heat will evaporate water from between hair fibres (capillary water) and from inside hair (internal water). It is internal water that is crucial for style achievement, as removing this water will create hydrogen bonds between neighbouring protein chains, effectively temporarily locking the desired style in place. The more water that is evaporated (i.e. the higher the temperature or the longer hair is dried for), the stronger these hydrogen bond links will be and the longer the style will last. Of course during water evaporation, hair has to be styled in the final shape, which is what curling tongs or flat irons do effectively by either creating a curl or straightening while heating (Fig. 3.29a, b).

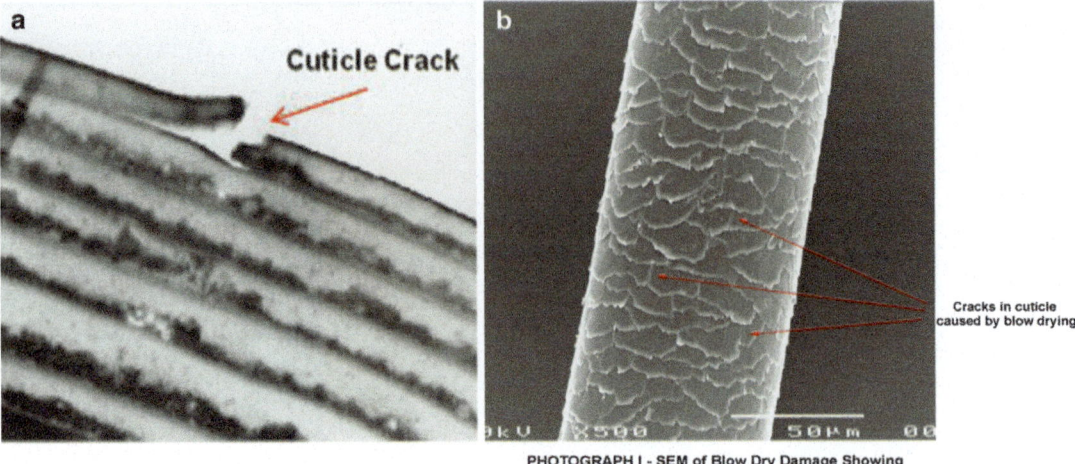

PHOTOGRAPH I - SEM of Blow Dry Damage Showing Cuticle Lifting and Cuticle Cracks

Fig. 3.30 Damage from blow drying: (**a**) cuticle cracks; (**b**) SEM image of cracks and cuticle lifting

Blow dryers are the most common form of heat used in the USA, and ~50 % of women use a blow dryer regularly. The air flow temperature is typically up to 100 °C, but hair will only get close to this temperature once capillary and internal water has evaporated. While hair is wet, heat will be absorbed by water while it is evaporating. No significant changes to the hair structure occur at these temperatures, but physical cracking of cuticles can occur at these temperatures if hair is dried very rapidly. These cracks occur as the rapidly drying cuticle contracts around a still-swollen cuticle. Once cracks are formed, the cuticle is more easily removed by combing, etc. (Fig. 3.30a, b).

Chemical degradation of hair due to heat will only occur if hair is heated above 150 °C. These temperatures can readily occur if heated straightening or curling irons are regularly used. With these implements on the highest setting, hair can reach temperatures of above 220 °C, especially if sections of hair are repeatedly straightened or hair is only slowly pulled through the flat iron. In addition, a critical degradation of protein takes place above 190 °C, which will involve cystine disulphide bond breakage. At very high levels of exposure to this temperature, melting of keratin can even occur. For example, Fig. 3.31 shows severe keratin degradation and hair breakage when hair is flat ironed for 3 min at 210 °C.

These exposures are extreme and are unlikely to occur, but excessive heat damage can be seen in increased incidence of broken hair for some women who use high-heat implements on a regular basis. These broken fibres will then lead to poor shine and smoothness, directly indicating poor hair health (Fig. 3.32). However, used with care, heated implements can also be used to increase perception of healthy hair. Blow dryers and flat irons straighten and align hair, giving it shine and making it easier to comb. In addition, creating a good 'wet set' by removing internal water will increase resistance of style to humidity, thus reducing frizz.

Chemical Treatments

Chemical treatments are the leading cause of hair structure changes and ultimately hair damage, but they also drive dramatic changes to either colour (e.g. permanent colouring) or style (e.g. perming, straightening). Women accept the damage trade-offs for the desired benefits. Damage from these treatments is not just of a higher category, but since all chemical treatments result in a breakdown of hair's protein and lipid

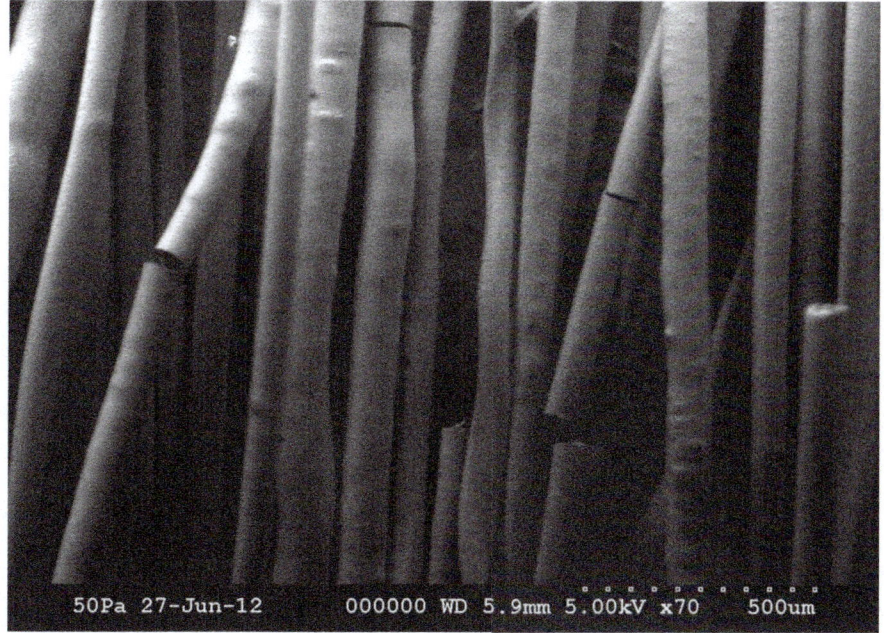

Fig. 3.31 Melted keratin and hair breakage caused by excessive heat of a flat iron

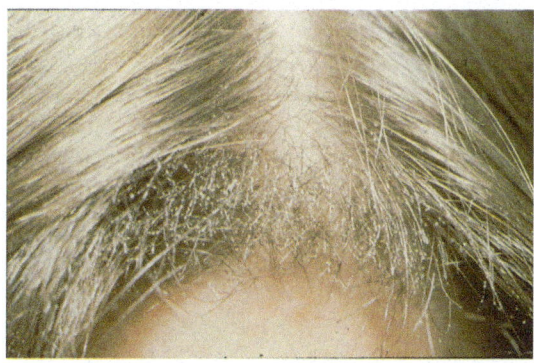

Fig. 3.32 Extreme variant of breakage

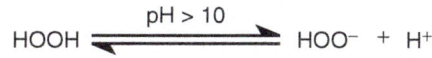

Fig. 3.33 Perhydroxyl anion (HOO⁻) is formed during the colouring process

Hair Colouring and Bleaching

Hair colouring is the most frequent chemical treatment worldwide. Forty percent of women colour their hair in the USA, 46 % in the UK, and 49 % in Japan (in past 3 months). It is increasing in popularity in large-population countries such as China, Brazil, and India.

The colouring process involves aggressive chemistry designed to lighten the hair by bleaching the natural pigment melanin and complex chemistry designed to form artificial colour within the hair. It is the combination of lightening and colour formation that gives the final shades, but it is the oxidant chemistry which is the main source of hair structure changes and, ultimately, hair damage.

There are two reactive species formed during the colouring process that have a significant impact on hair health via several mechanisms. The first species is the perhydroxyl anion (HOO⁻) which is formed from hydrogen peroxide and ammonia at the high pH used in colourants. This species is crucial for bleaching melanin so there is always a trade-off between colouring performance and damage caused (Fig. 3.33).

The perhydroxyl anion is responsible for two major chemistries that directly impact hair health.

structures, it renders hair more susceptible to subsequent damage from physical and heat processes. Women often will moderate their habits and practices once they start employing chemical treatments such as colouring by reducing washing frequencies and moderating heated implement temperatures.

$$\text{---S---S---} \longrightarrow \text{---SO}_3^- \quad {}^-\text{O}_3\text{S---}$$

Fig. 3.34 The second chemical effect that the perhydroxyl anion will perform is to break disulphide bonds of the cross-linking amino acid cystine to form cystic acid

The first is removal via perhydrolysis of the surface lipid layer (f-layer or 18-methyleicosanoic acid) that is present on each cuticle cell.

This lipid provides a protective hydrophobic coating which reduces friction forces, especially when hair is wet, and gives hair its smooth and soft feel. Once removed after colouring, the surface properties of hair dramatically change, with wet friction increasing significantly in addition to loss of soft hair feel and shine.

Once friction is increased, damage to hair from combing and brushing also significantly increases with an accelerated formation of knots and tangles. This additional damage can be reduced with use of conditioners, but removal of the hydrophobic lipid layer also has a consequence of reducing deposition levels of conditioning actives, especially silicones. Over the last few years, this chemistry has been well explored, and strategies to reduce the impact of surface lipid removal via colouring have been introduced. There has been an explosion in the identification of new silicone materials that will have an improved deposition profile on coloured hair.

The second chemical effect that the perhydroxyl anion will perform is to break disulphide bonds of the cross-linking amino acid cystine to form cystic acid (Fig. 3.34). As a consequence of this breakage, the tensile strength of hair is decreased, and increased protein degradation and loss after washing can be measured. Women will potentially notice this as increased breakage, especially at hair tips, where hair may have been exposed to several colouring treatments.

The second reactive species is the highly reactive hydroxyl radical (HO*), which is formed during the reaction of hydrogen peroxide and any low levels of metals such as copper and iron that are present on hair. In most cases, this is an unwanted side reaction that can be avoided by use of specific products, e.g. products that contain chelants which specifically target any copper in hair and prevent formation of highly reactive hydroxyl radicals. This chemistry is catalytic, i.e. low levels of copper will generate multiple hydroxyl radicals. Hydroxy radicals will not specifically target any part of hair but will react with both proteins and lipids, causing degradation of these structures and ultimately leading to easier breakdown with combing, brushing, etc.

All hair types will be impacted in a similar way, but women using lighter shades such as extra-light blondes will generally have more damage, mainly driven by higher levels of hydrogen peroxide used to achieve the lighter shades.

Hair damage may be lower for women colouring in the salon vs. at home, not because of different chemistry being used but due to more skilled application methods. In the salon, the stylist will apply colour to hair roots on the regrowth followed either by applying the same colour to remaining hair for the last 10–15 min of total treatment time or using a lower hydrogen peroxide shade on the mid and tips. At home, women may inadvertently apply colour over the whole head, giving a less even colour and more cumulative damage.

Hair damage is significantly higher if women are looking for a more significant shade transition from dark to light and hair bleaches are used. These bleaches typically come as powders that contain persulphate salts and silicates to provide alkalinity. These are mixed with hydrogen peroxide, forming chemistry that will significantly bleach melanin in dark hair or preformed dyes. The mechanism of bleaching is via formation of highly reactive free radicals which do an efficient job of bleaching melanin, but also cause damage to keratin, leading to loss of tensile strength and also making hair vulnerable to subsequent combing and brushing damage (Fig. 3.35a, b). Typically, hair damage is minimised by only using this chemistry for highlights (i.e. only selected strands) or applying for newly grown roots.

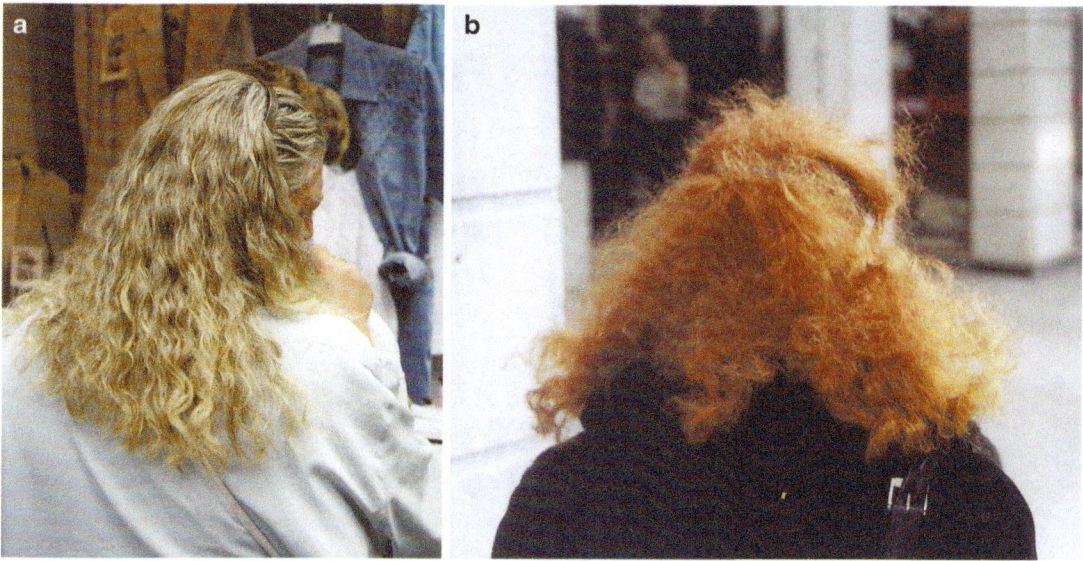

Fig. 3.35 The mechanism of bleaching is via formation of highly reactive free radicals which do an efficient job of (**a**) bleaching melanin, but also (**b**) cause damage to keratin

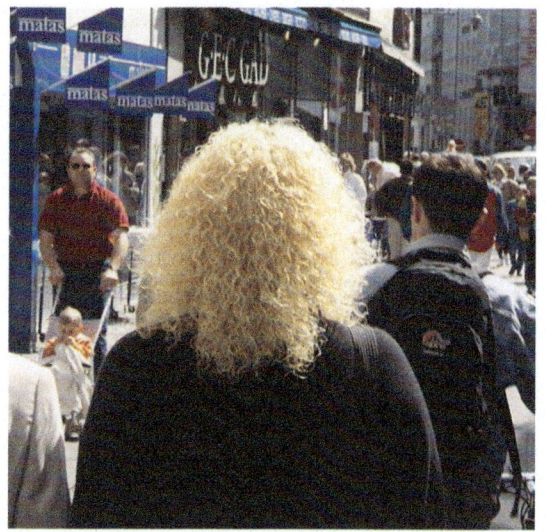

Fig. 3.36 Results of perming

Perming

The incidence of perming in some countries such as the USA and UK is relatively low (~10 %), but it is higher in Asian countries such as Japan (~20 %). The majority of perms are performed by stylists because the risk of damage from these treatments can be high. The chemistry involves breaking of cystine disulphide bonds, typically with thioglycolic acid, followed by arrangement of hair into a desired configuration, then reforming the disulphide bonds with hydrogen peroxide setting the style in place. The bond reforming is not 100 % effective, so internal strength will always be reduced by these treatments. In addition, hair types will respond to perming chemistry differently. Consequently, there is no fixed time for the initial bond breaking stage. Stylists are skilled to stop the chemistry before the hair structure is severely compromised. In situations where excess chemistry is used, hair will become easy to break, and additional broken fibres will be noticed after treatments (Fig. 3.36).

Straightening and Relaxing

Over the last few years, permanent hair straightening for women with slight to moderate curl levels has become more popular, mainly driven by products such as Brazilian keratin treatments (BKT), which use actives such as formaldehyde to cross-link keratins in hair to 'lock-in' the straight style. There have been safety concerns raised about the use of formaldehyde and methylene glycol, which has led to new chemistries appearing on the market (e.g. glyoxylic acid).

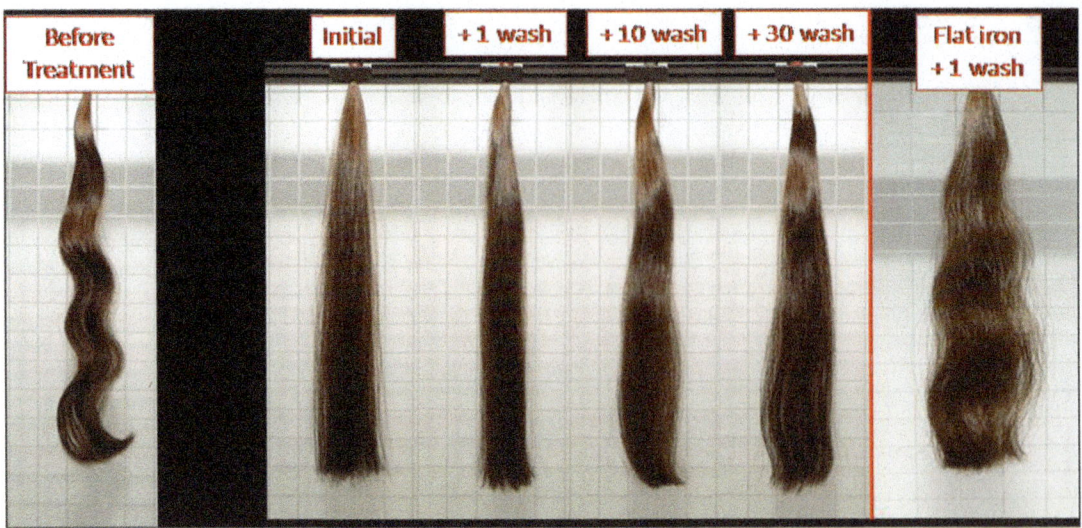

Fig. 3.37 Lab test of Brazilian keratin treatment (BKT), from initial results to noticeable decrease in straightening due to subsequent washings

The process for these treatments is to diffuse the cross-linking active into hair and then activate cross-linking chemistry using heat while setting hair into the desired shape using a flat iron.

A recent study by Dr. J. Marsh and Dr. M. Gavazzoni examined the effects on performance over time after the application of a BKT that contains formaldehyde as a cross-linking agent. Figure 3.37 illustrates that there are initial excellent aesthetic results, which decrease with washing frequency.

In many cases, women will refer to hair health benefits deriving from such treatments where these benefits are driven by the macroscopic results—straight vs. wavy or curly hair. The first is higher alignment of straight vs. wavy hair, which will improve shine and offer a smoother feel. The second is a frizz improvement, where hair remains in its straight shape even at high humidity in comparison to wavy hair, which will return to its wavy/frizz configuration. However, in some cases, breakage after repeated treatments has been noticed. This is driven in part by the flat-ironing high heat used to achieve the final shape.

Another chemistry used for straightening is thioglycolate to break disulphides and hydrogen peroxide to reset in the new straight shape. This chemistry is the same as used in perming and has the same risks of overprocessing. The hair health benefits that come from a straight style are higher in this case than for women choosing to add curls. This is due to reduced incidence of knot formation, tangles, increased alignment, and shine and decreased frizz.

The above two treatments are suitable for women who have low to moderate levels of curl, but not for highly curled or coiled hair such as women of African descent.

In this latter case, more aggressive chemistry is required to restructure hair, and with this comes significantly higher levels of damage. Relaxing treatments designed to do this use very high alkalinity (>pH 13) with sodium hydroxide (lye relaxers) or guanidine hydroxide (non-lye relaxers) to more efficiently break disulphide bonds and eventually form lanthionine bridges in the straightened shape. As with perms, there is a danger of overprocessing with this chemistry, leading to very high breakage, and even if used by skilled stylists, there will be some breakage observed. Women who regularly relax their hair need to take great care not to cause excessive breakage by regularly using oil treatments and minimising wash frequency and heat exposure.

Combination of chemical treatments and physical processes can also drive significantly higher cuticle abrasion and breakage due to a number of factors. The first is removal of the hydrophobic f-layer lipid on the cuticle surface by chemical treatments such as colouring and highlighting, leaving a surface that is more hydrophilic. This increases frictional forces and also reduces deposition of conditioning actives such as silicones which can reduce these frictional forces (i.e. the protection benefit of conditioning products decreases). The second is reduction in tensile strength of hair, making breakage more likely. This is especially the case for treatments which involve a significant amount of bond breakage, such as perming and relaxing treatments, which rely on breaking cystine to straighten hair.

Minimising Damage

The fortunate few who have a growing phase (anagen) sufficient to produce hair long enough to sit on may have tips which have survived for 7 or 8 years. Throughout its growth, this hair tip needs to be cared for to keep its 'healthy' look as manifest by shine and manageability. A damaged cuticle cannot heal, although much can be done to help its appearance.

Common sense dictates that hair cleaned frequently, using good-quality products and—most importantly—being conditioned, is the bedrock of hair care. Regular trimming of the ends by a skilled stylist to prevent weathering effects such as split ends is to be encouraged (Fig. 3.38), and a 'good' cut is the basis of the desired style (see Chap. 5).

Changing hair colour requires advice from an experienced hair technician, who can advise on how much colour change a particular hair can stand and which hair-colouring products would be suitable. With an understanding of the principles of good hair care, and regularly putting those principles into practice, everyone can aim to keep their hair in good condition.

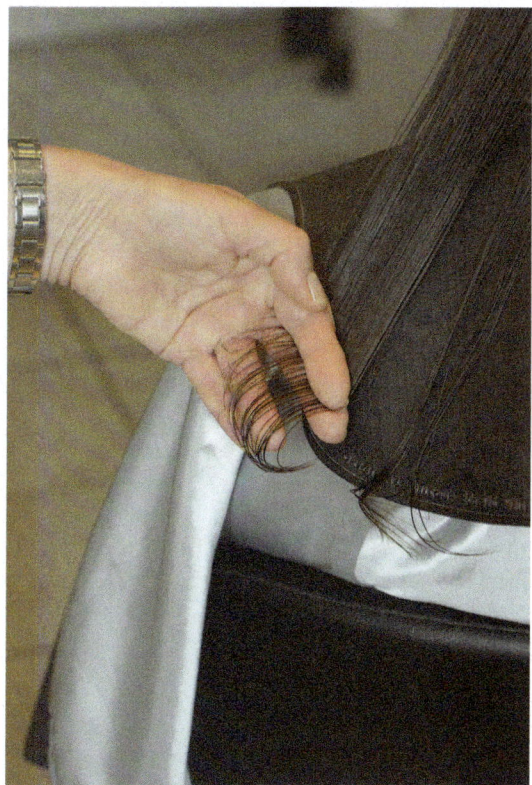

Fig. 3.38 Regular trimming of the hair ends by a skilled stylist, to prevent weathering effects such as split ends, is encouraged

General Principles

The natural look of hair depends on several factors. Hair that is in poor condition looks dull and dry. The presence or absence of natural oils makes a difference, and very straight hair reflects light better than tousled hair does.

Inevitably, trying to improve upon nature, not just once but over and over again, leads to many pitfalls, which includes:

- Not understanding the basic properties of hair in general and one's own hair in particular.
- Trying to lighten the colour of hair more than it can stand (bleach damage).
- Continually trying to correct previous mistakes.

It is all too easy to fall into the trap of blaming the last product put onto the hair as the single cause of a problem. More often, hair condition is lost as a result of a combination of mistreatments over a long period.

Once significantly damaged, the cuticle cannot be repaired, and hair care must be aimed at preventing injury in the first place. All procedures should be carried out as gently as possible. Apart from this, the best way to keep damage to a minimum is to condition regularly and thoroughly. This helps to keep the cuticle intact, lower friction, and reduce static charge on the hair.

In the next chapter, a senior dermatologist explains the major problems encountered with hair and hair health before we consider some of the cosmetic solutions in Chap. 5.

References

1. Thibaut S, De Becker E, Bernard BA, Huart M, Fiat F, Baghdadli N, et al. Chronological ageing of human hair keratin fibres. Int J Cosmet Sci. 2010;32(6):422–34.
2. Fink B, Neuser F, Deloux G, Röder S, Matts PJ. Visual attention to and perception of undamaged and damaged versions of natural and colored female hair. J Cosmet Dermatol. 2013;12:78–84.
3. Marsh JM, Iveson R, Flagler MJ, Davis MG, Newland AB, Greiss KD, et al. Role of copper in photochemical damage to hair. Int J Cosmet Sci. 2014;36(1):32–8.
4. Pande CM, Albrecht L, Yang B. Hair photoprotection by dyes. Int J Cosmet Sci. 2001;52:377–89.
5. Naqvi KR, Marsh JM, Godfrey S, Davis MG, Flagler MJ, Hao J, et al. The role of chelants in controlling Cu(II)-induced radical chemistry in oxidative hair colouring products. Int J Cosmet Sci. 2013;35(1):41–9.

Healthy Hair Method Assessments

Introduction

There is perhaps a misconception that hair-care products are mere commodities of a simplistic nature: technologically limited and lacking the sophistication of skin-care products. Nothing, in fact, could be further from the truth. As stated by one of the world's leading authorities in hair care, Dr. Rodney Dawber, Emeritus Clinical Reader at Oxford, 'Shampoos represent the ultimate in simplicity from complexity. A product everyone can use anywhere, any when, and expect to achieve the same result'.

To achieve this, the cosmetic scientist and the major cosmetic companies spend years and millions of dollars in research to bring products to the global market. These products address the needs of modern women (and men) with differing hair phenotypes and different habits and practices in their personal regimens (Fig. 4.1).

As part of this research and development programme, the cosmetic scientist needs to be able to assess the substrate (the hair) and measure the effect of hair-care products. There are many such methods published in the literature and which are utilised by the cosmetic industry. Invariably, these are performed in the laboratory on pre-prepared samples of hair, known as tresses. These tresses are meticulously assembled from either a single donor (such as in pure blonde hair—one of the most valuable commodities on the planet) or a composite from different donors. Hairs are inspected for signs of damage; quality is assured, and hairs are assembled in a tress in a precise root-to-tip direction. This ensures reproducible investigation of the efficacy of any hair-care product tested (Fig. 4.2).

Women in real life, however, use various and unquantifiable signals to assess how healthy their hair is. This will be a combination of feel when dry and wet and how easily styling is to achieve and retain and, most importantly, how shiny hair appears.

Hair stylists are often more sensitive to hair health differences due to their experience with a wide range of hair types. Typically, however, their assessment will be made at a single point in time when women are at the salon (Fig. 4.3). In general, both women and hairstylists can predict their hair health quite accurately using a variety of so-called touch points as shown in Fig. 4.4a–e.

Despite the sophistication of methodologies and technologies available to the cosmetic scientist, it is unlikely that one scientific method will, alone, be sufficient to correlate with this consumer and stylist perception. As a result, a series of strategies to assess hair health have been developed.

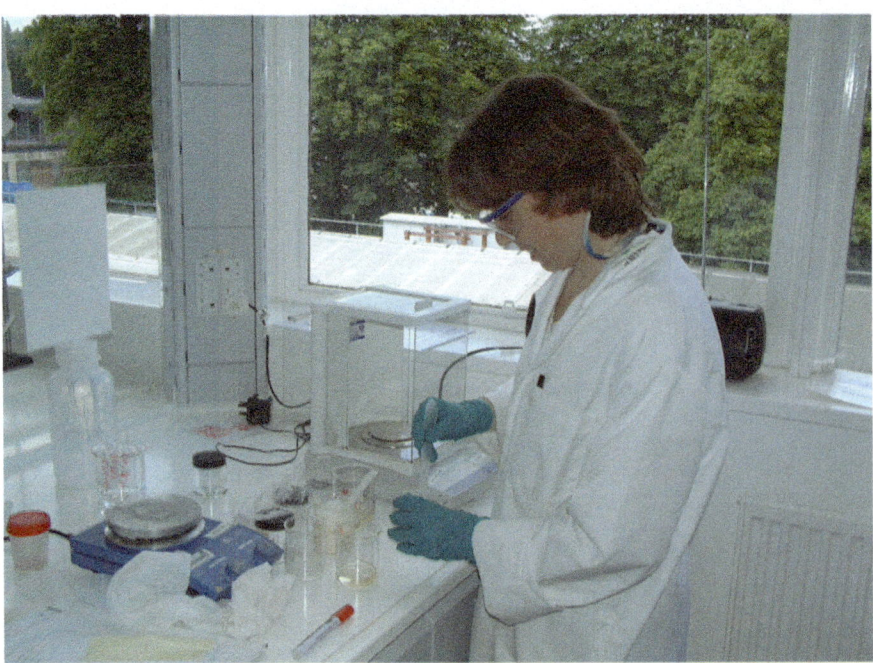

Fig. 4.1 The cosmetic scientist and the major cosmetic companies spend years and millions of dollars in research to bring products to the global market. Courtesy Dr. Jennifer Marsh, PhD

Fig. 4.2 A hair tress being prepared to test the efficacy of a hair-care product

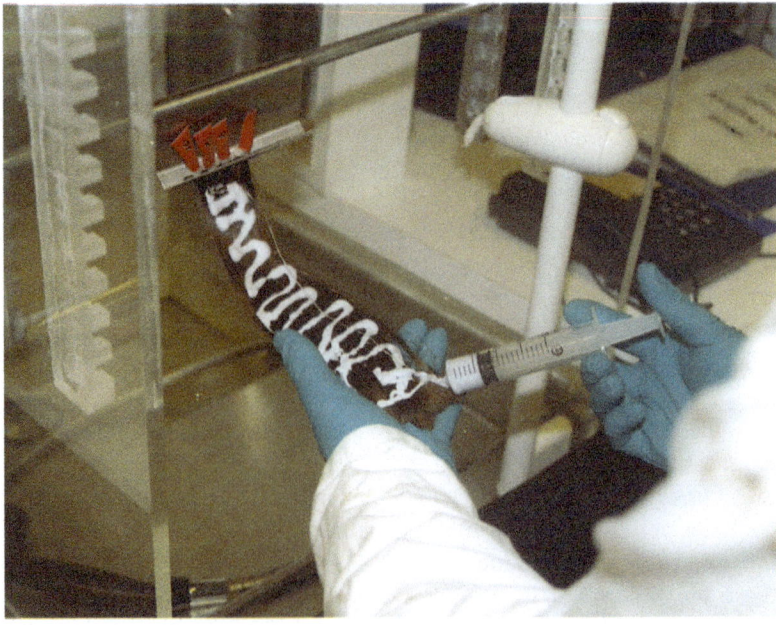

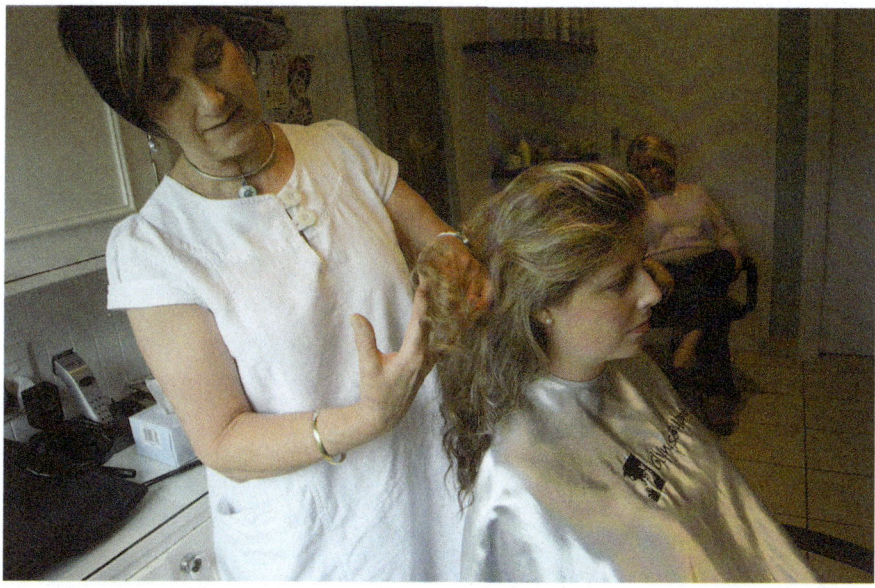

Fig. 4.3 Hairstylists are often more sensitive to hair health differences due to their experience with a wide range of hair types

Multiple Strategies to Assess Hair Health

The cosmetic scientist employs a range of strategies and, within these, various techniques or methodologies in order to be able to quantify the different touch points that women use to assess hair health:

- **Strategy 1**: This first set of methodologies is designed to mimic how a woman assesses a particular health aspect of a product, for example, creating shine or reducing combing force. Typically, these methods use bulk hair arrays, and care is taken to create hair tresses that can reliably reproduce a product performance profile mimicking the experience by women.
- **Strategy 2**: The second set of methods investigates single fibre properties, particularly, how these properties are impacted by UV exposure or chemical treatments. Other examples include mechanical properties of the hair such as tensile strength and structural changes such as cuticle damage.
- **Strategy 3**: The third set of methods investigates the structural changes to hair at the micro level, often measuring specific changes to proteins or lipid degradation. This strategy results in a mechanistic understanding of how the hair structure is being altered by the various damaging insults to which it is exposed. These can then be linked back to both the single fibre property changes and the bulk array property changes in order to explain how these changes manifest themselves in a way relevant to women.
- **Strategy 4**: The fourth set of methods assesses the health of the follicle and its relationship to the hair quality as it grows from the scalp. These methods are important to assess possible disease states and to determine likely susceptibility of hair to external insults as it grows.

Figure 4.5 illustrates the full array of hair health methods. In addition, some of these aspects are discussed in Chap. 5.

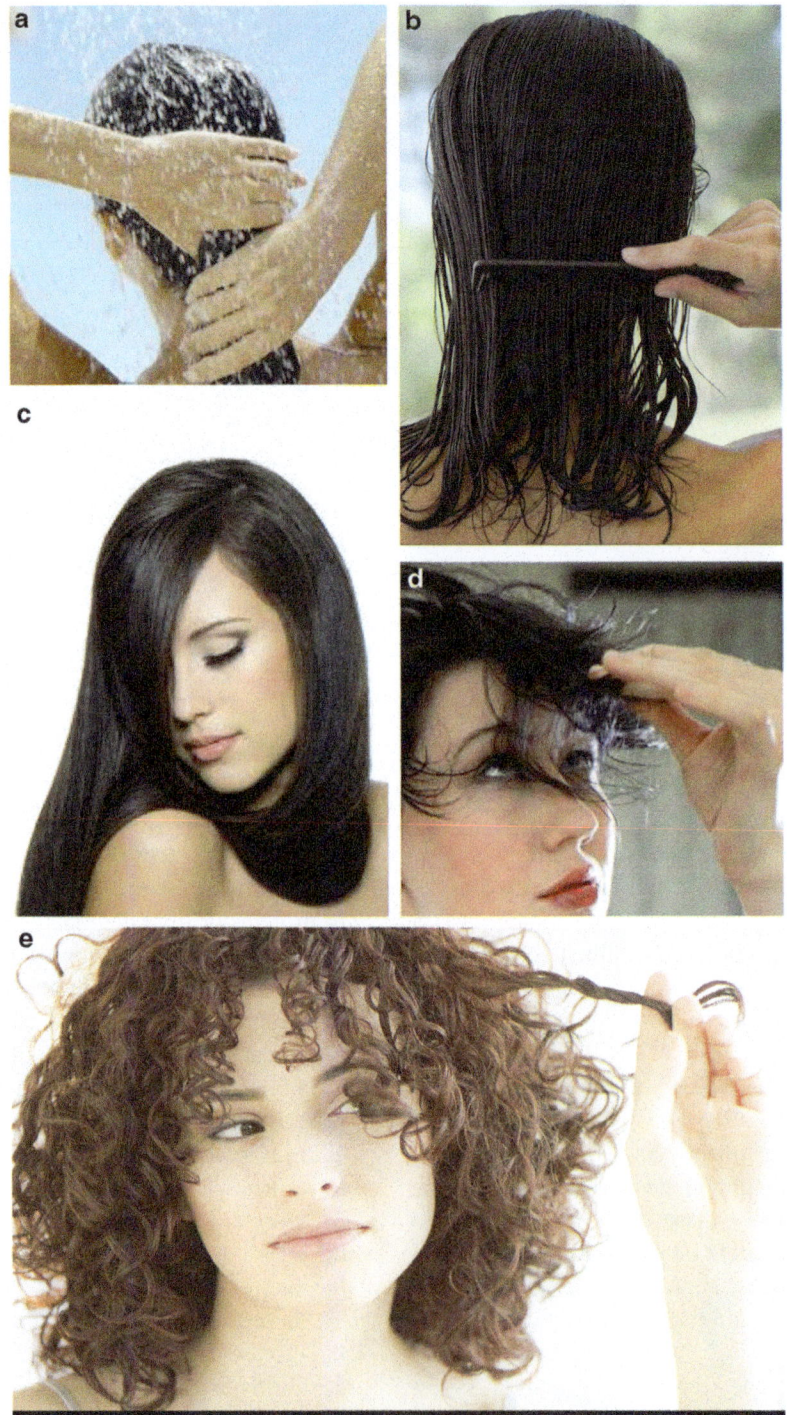

Fig. 4.4 Multiple touch points used by women and stylists to predict hair health—feel and look of hair when (**a**, **b**) wet and (**c**–**e**) dry

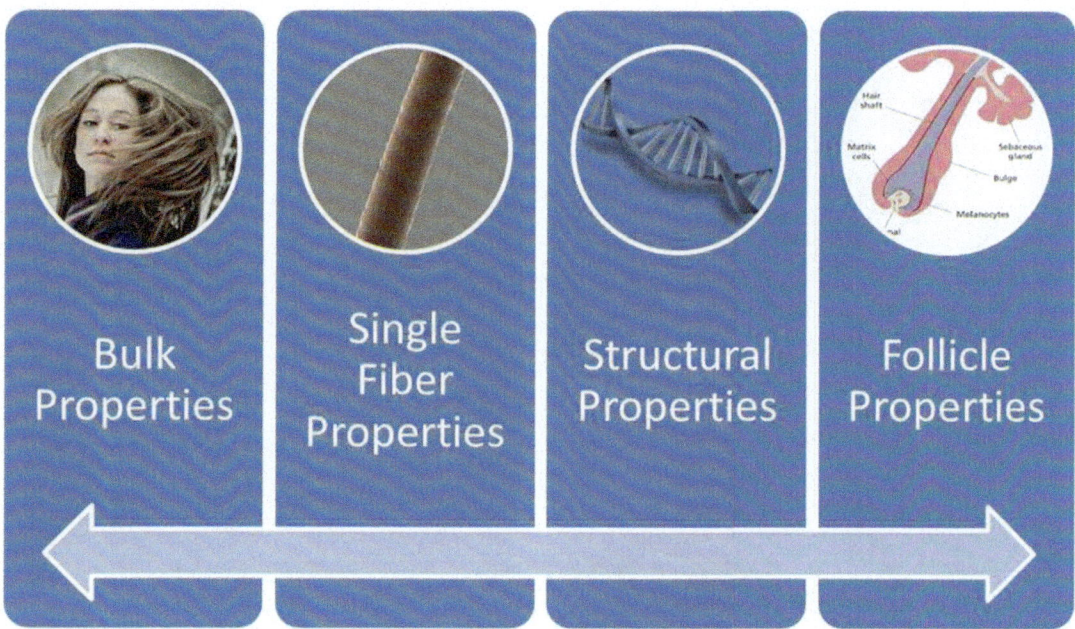

Fig. 4.5 The full array of hair health methods

Strategy 1: Assessment of Hair (Self or Observer)

To assess one's own hair health or that of another, there are several pieces of information that may enable this process. First is a visual examination of the hair—is it fine or coarse, straight or curly, long or short? Does it have a good style and look shiny and is well aligned? Does it look smooth, or are broken fibres present?

The second aspect is the feel of the hair—do the tips feel very different from the roots, does it feel rough or smooth? Careful examination of the tips may reveal split ends. There may be a dramatic colour difference from root to tip (folding the hair tips back to the scalp assists in the assessment). If the hair is long enough, gathering up the hair into a ponytail and feeling (and observing) how full it seems and how much it narrows at the tips may be useful (Figs. 4.6, 4.7, 4.8, and 4.9).

If this assessment is being carried out as part of a research study, a series of questions which

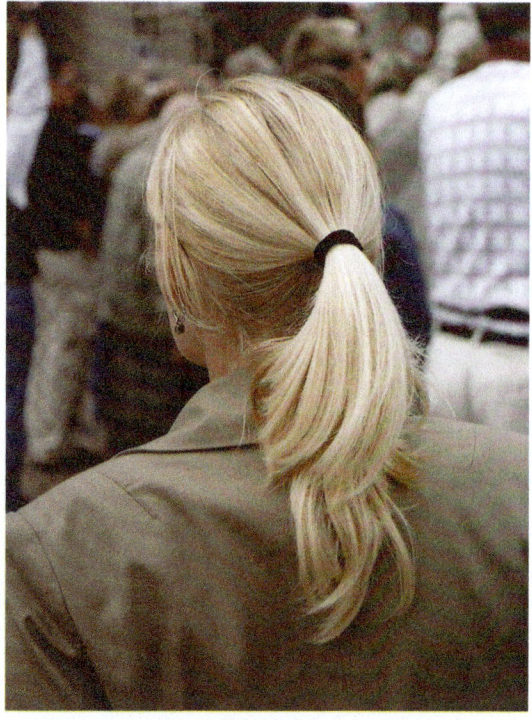

Fig. 4.6 Thick ponytail despite UV bleaching

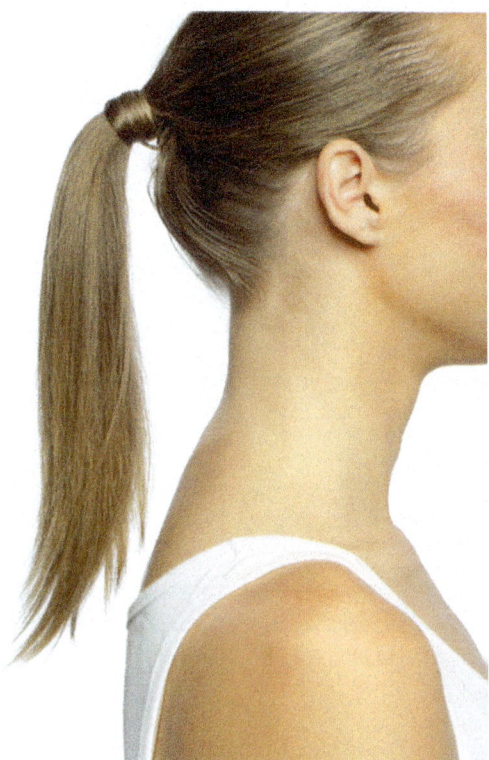

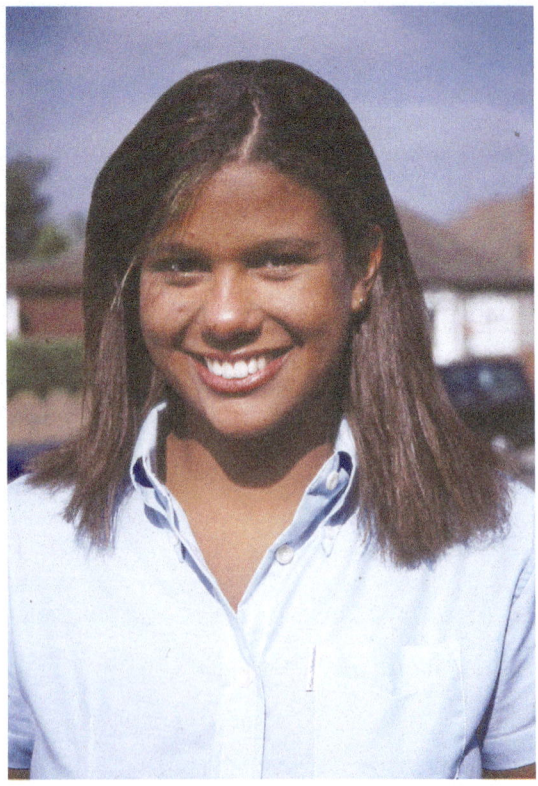

Fig. 4.7 Thinning ponytail due to excessive weathering and breakage

Fig. 4.8 Colour difference from root to tip due to repeated chemical straightening

probe the frequency and severity of any insults to which hair is exposed should be made. These include chemical treatments, sun exposure, heat implement usage, wash frequency, etc. A review should also be made of any products that are being used to protect hair, such as deep conditioning treatments and heat protection sprays.

This strategy results in the creation of Table 4.1, which highlights some key activities and their relative contribution to hair damage, either to create damage or prevent damage. Some treatments are more likely to create damage, and this is reflected in the chart.

Instrumental Methods

In this section, a selection of methods in each category is described which act as an illustration of key methods of assessment used routinely in the cosmetics industry.

The main objective behind instrumental methods is to design a test that can measure differences in hair properties that are important to hair health such as shine, combing force, hair feel, etc.

To achieve this, care is taken to ensure reproducibility of hair source and size of hair tresses. In many cases, hair from multiple women is first screened for low to moderate damage levels and then blended to create a uniform substrate (Fig. 4.10).

Care is taken to keep the method as close as possible to how women would treat their hair. As an example, the combing speed in an automated combing force test is close to the speed used by women.

Assessment of Shine

Shine is a complex property to measure and is exceptionally difficult to fully correlate to consumer perception. The main issue is that women do not just use visual cues to assess shine but also use feel cues, most noticeably softness. A common response to how shiny a woman finds her hair is the running of fingers through the hair. If it

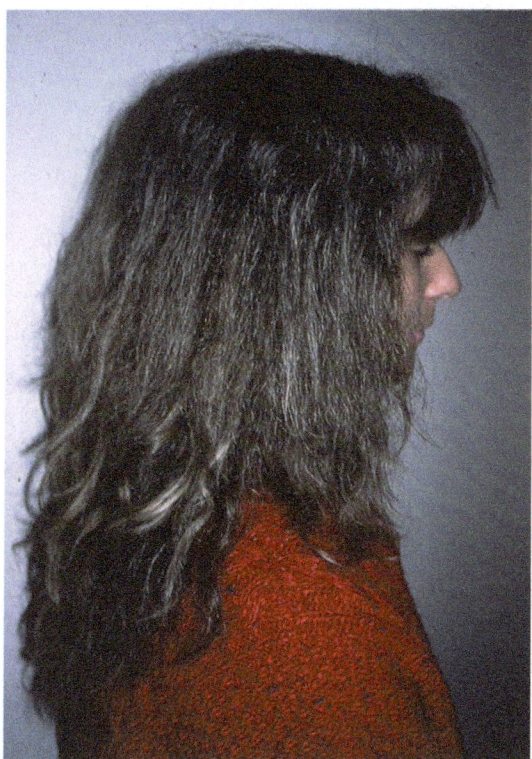

Fig. 4.9 Split ends clearly visible

Table 4.1 Scoring system for hair damage

	More than every 6 weeks	Every 6 weeks to 3 months	Less than every 3 months
Bleaching	+10 pts	+5 pts	+1 pt
Perming	+10 pts	+5 pts	+1 pt
Colouring	+10 pts	+5 pts	+1 pt
Hair cut	−3 pts	−2 pts	−1 pt

	More than 5 × a week	Between 1 × per week and 5 × per week	Less than once per week
Flat iron	+5 pts	+3 pts	+1 pt
Blow dry	+3 pts	+2 pts	+1 pt
Combing/brushing	+3 pts	+2 pts	+1 pt
Washing	+3 pts	+2 pts	+1 pt
Deep conditioning treatment	−5 pts	−3 pts	−1 pt
Rinse off conditioner	−3 pts	−2 pts	−1 pt
Heat protection spray	−3 pts	−2 pts	−1 pt

	More than 5 h per day	1–5 h per day	Less than 5 h per day
Sun exposure	+5 pts	+3 pts	+1 pt

High hair damage	Medium hair damage	Low hair damage
>18 pts	<18 pts, >7 pts	<7 pts

hair strand and be either absorbed or reflected from the back surface of hair through the hair strand again and back out to the eye to give the chroma reflection. The intensity of the chroma reflection will depend on hair colour (darker hair = less chroma reflection), and it is offset from the front-side reflection due to the cuticle pitch (Fig. 4.12). This chroma band gives hair its natural appearance unlike, for example, nylon strands or artificial hair.

Instrumentation has been developed to measure these light interactions with hair. Several algorithms have been developed to convert collected data into 'shine' values. Because alignment is such an overwhelming driver of shine perception, measurements can either be made with aligned or non-aligned tresses depending on the information that is required.

In an aligned configuration, hair tresses are mounted onto a rounded surface. A beam of light is directed at the hair under controlled lighting conditions. Hair tresses are imaged with a digital camera and analysed by calculating diffuse reflection, specular reflection, chroma reflection, and width of the combined specular/chroma peak (Fig. 4.13) [1].

The surface of the hair determines what happens to light reflection. A virgin hair has a relatively smooth cuticle. Heavily damaged hair may have gross disruption, and this interferes with reflection, thus giving lower shine.

Combing, Frictional Forces, and Breakage

These methods all ultimately can be related to hair health properties such as smooth feel and breakage, and all are often used to measure the efficacy of conditioning products designed to increase

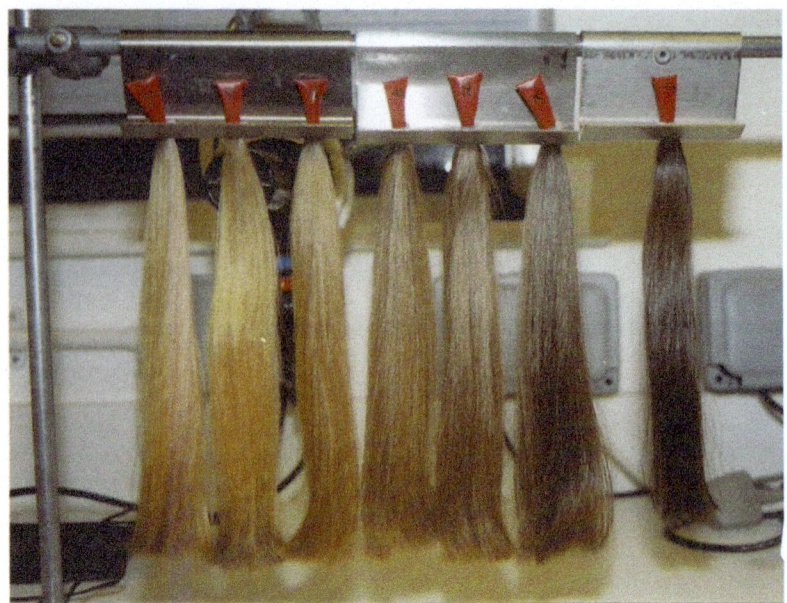

Fig. 4.10 Care is taken to ensure reproducibility of hair source and size of hair tresses. In many cases, hair from multiple women is first screened for low to moderate damage levels and then blended to create a uniform substrate

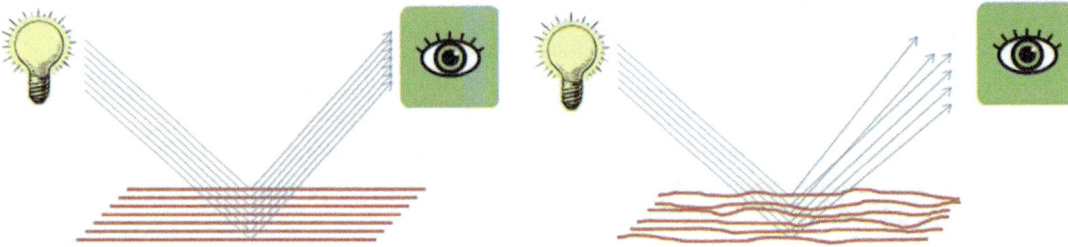

Fig. 4.11 Comparison of high and low shine

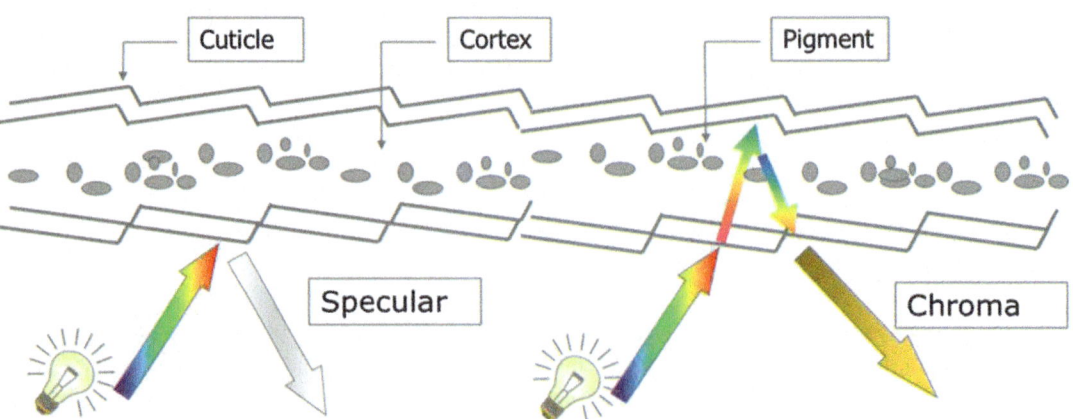

Fig. 4.12 Specular and chroma reflection

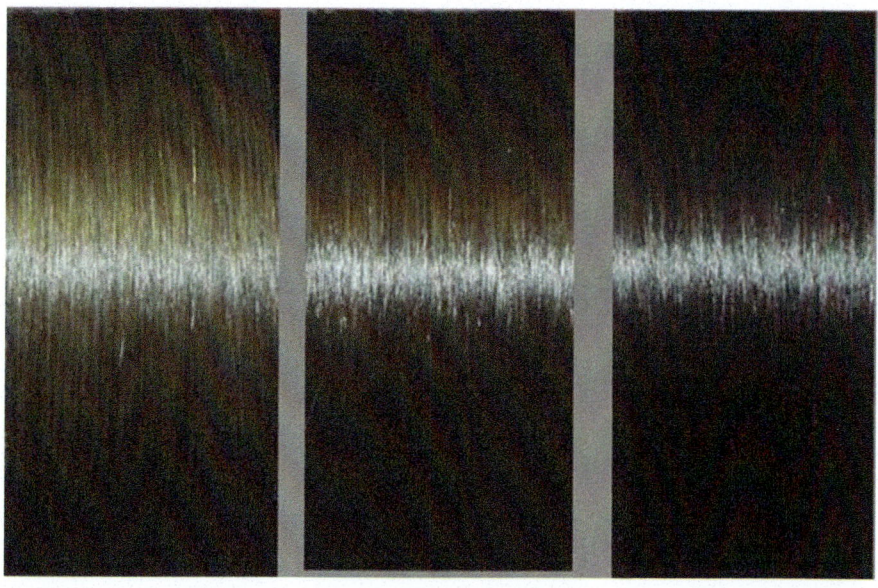

Fig. 4.13 Reflection differences from three variants of brown hair. From *left* to *right*: light, medium, and dark

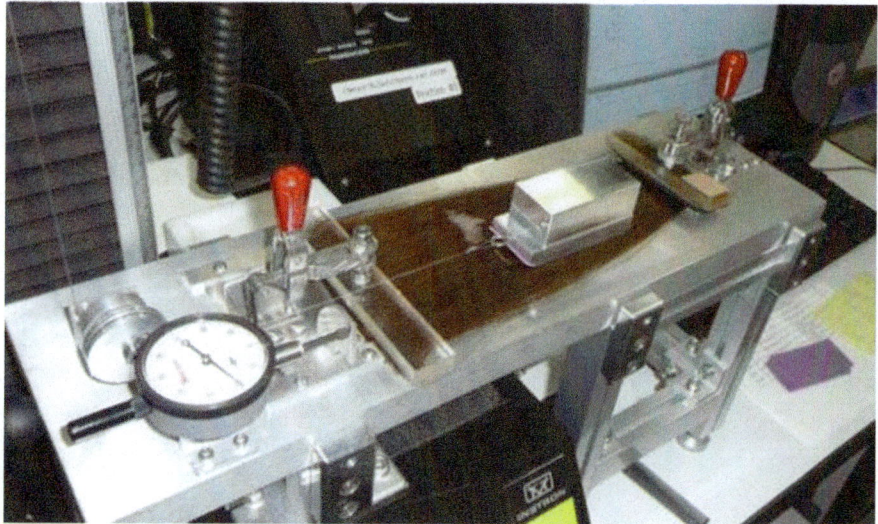

Fig. 4.14 Measuring frictional forces

lubrication between strands. Assessment of combing forces is a standard method in the hair-care industry and involves a sensitive instrument that measures the force required to pull hair through either one or two static combs. It can be performed with either wet or dry hair, and in both cases, the tresses are detangled before measurement.

Frictional forces are measured as the force required to move an object across the hair surface under a constant speed. Again, either wet or dry tresses can be used, but typically dry measurements are more commonly made (Fig. 4.14).

Breakage is measured on tresses using repeated combing and then measuring either weight loss from the initial tress or collecting and weighing broken fibres. Automated combing wheels have been designed to standardise the combing process and make the tests easier to perform (Fig. 4.15a–c).

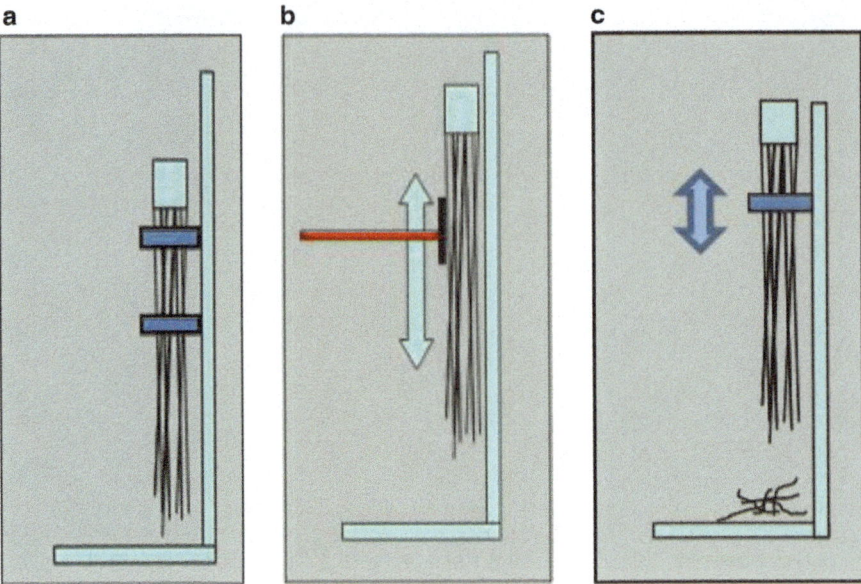

Fig. 4.15 Schematic of hair measurements: (**a**) combing measurements; (**b**) friction measurements; (**c**) breakage measurements

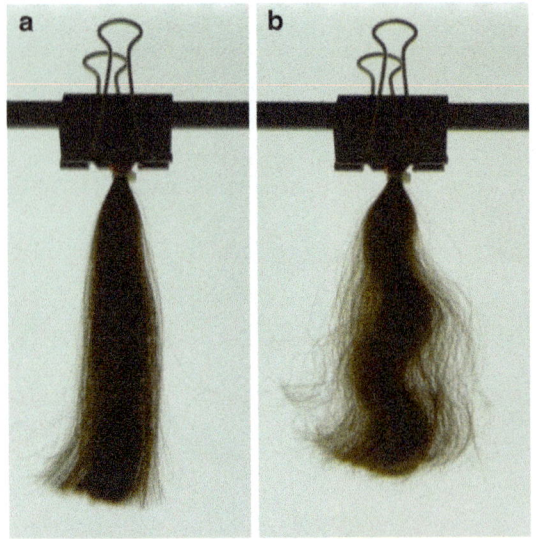

Fig. 4.16 Frizz image assessment at (**a**) low and (**b**) high relative humidity

Frizz

Frizz is typically measured by assessing expansion of hair after it has been set into a style in a low-humidity environment (e.g. 20 % relative humidity [RH]) and then moved to a high-humidity environment (e.g. 80 % RH). The assessment of expansion can be visual or by images captured and analysed for parameters such as total tress area or width increase (Fig. 4.16a, b). This methodology can be used to assess the efficacy of conditioning products designed to reduce frizz.

Strategy 2: Single Fibre Mechanical Properties

Breakage, volume, and manageability, all of these properties depend strongly on fibre dimensions (diameter and ellipticity). Accordingly, values will vary widely from fibre to fibre. To more accurately measure the intrinsic mechanical properties and remove the influence of fibre dimension, the diameter is typically measured for each fibre and the mechanical properties expressed as a modulus (e.g. a force to break per unit area). In this manner, the influence of different treatments and insults may be more accurately compared.

As seen in Fig. 4.17, the three important single fibre mechanical properties are tensile (force to stretch), torsion (force to twist), and bending (force to bend). The most common single fibre mechanical property measured is the tensile strength, as it is most closely related to perception of hair strength. Typically, a single fibre is pulled under constant force until it breaks to create the force-extension curve shown in Fig. 4.18. Different parameters can be calculated from these curves, but the most important are Young's modulus (slope of initial elastic region), plateau load, break force, and break extension. These parameters can be measured with either wet or dry hair depending on the type of treatment used. This curve will change with wet hair vs. dry hair because hair is more easily stretched and broken when wet. The slope of the Young's modulus will decrease and the break force point will be reached at a lower extension. In addition, the curve will change as a function of chemical treatments, especially if hair is severely damaged.

Visualising Damage

It is often helpful to visualise damage to hair using high-magnification image methods. These methods are infrequently quantitative but, when used in combination with other methods, do give insights into what is driving numerical differences. Two key methods in this area are scanning electron microscopy (SEM) and transmission electron microscopy (TEM). SEM is typically used to assess surface deposition or cuticle quality. TEM is typically used to assess cuticle and cortical structural features in cross sections.

Shown in Figs. 4.19a, b and 4.20a, b are images of the root and tip of a hair in SEM and TEM from a woman with damaged hair (e.g. a regular colourer and heat implement user).

Strategy 3: Structural Property Measures

It is often insightful to directly measure changes to the hair's structure in order to understand the fundamental mechanism and to provide an objective method to assess the effect of hair-care

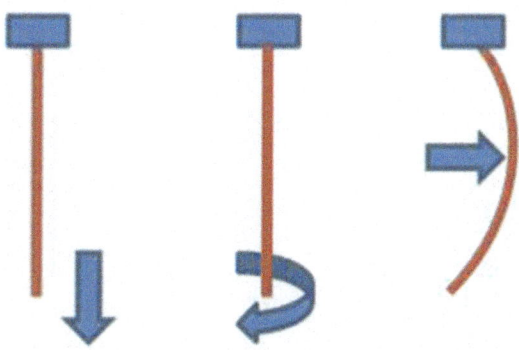

Fig. 4.17 The three important single fibre mechanical properties are from *left* to *right*, tensile (force to stretch), torsion (force to twist), and bending (force to bend)

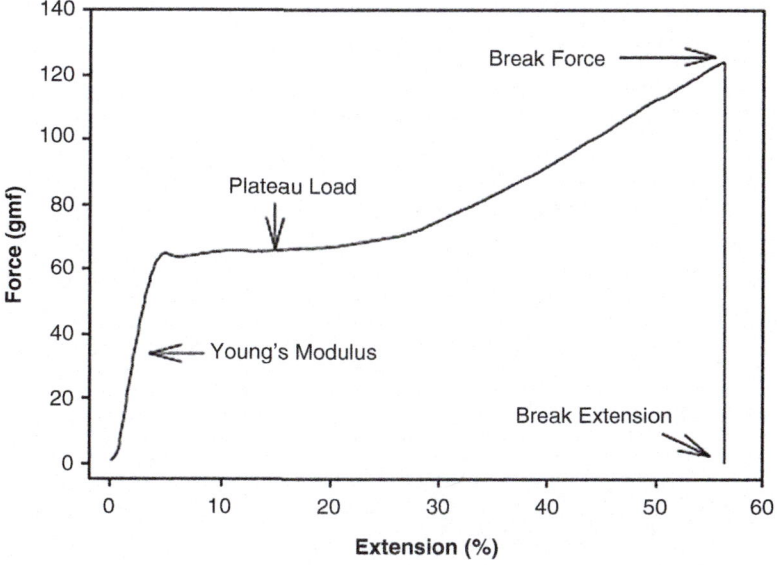

Fig. 4.18 Tensile profile of hair

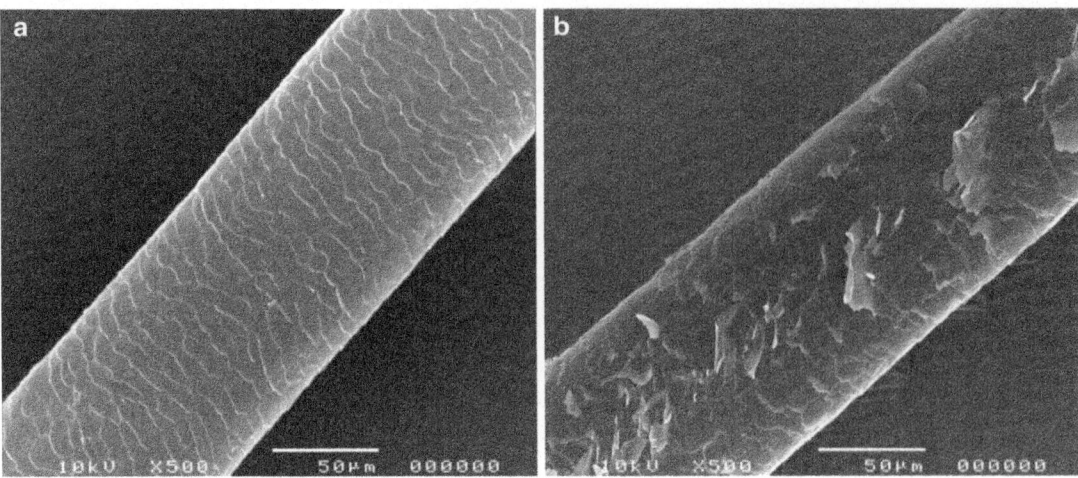

Fig. 4.19 Scanning electron microscopy (SEM) images of (**a**) root and (**b**) tip

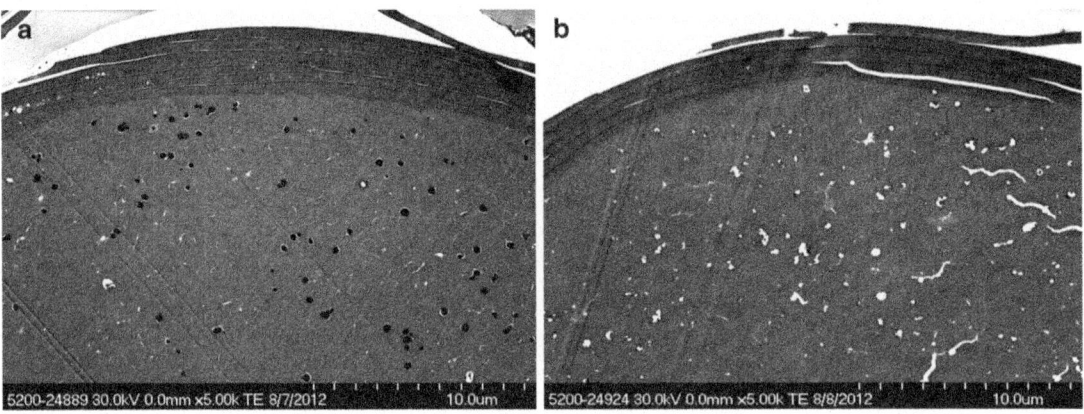

Fig. 4.20 Transmission electron microscope (TEM) images of (**a**) root and (**b**) tip

products. These measures include the changes to protein or lipid structures compared to the consequences of these changes. An example is how break force is impacted or how shine is reduced.

The methods are often more sensitive than measuring bulk or single fibre properties and give mechanistic insights as to how different types of insults impact on hair health properties. As a prime example, oxidative colouring removes the surface bound lipid (f-layer) from hair via a perhydrolysis mechanism. It is possible to directly measure this particular lipid and demonstrate its reduction after colouring and measure its impact on combing and friction forces. The combing force and friction measurements are more relevant to how women will refer to colouring damage, but the direct measures relate to the mechanisms driving these perceptions.

Protein Changes in the Hair Shaft

The assessment of protein changes within the hair shaft has proved to be one of the most important assessments of response to various insults. A relatively simple test in this area is the measurement of the protein fragments produced after shaking hair in water for a defined period of time (viz. one hour). The total protein derived from this procedure can be measured by different assays including Lowry assay and Bradford assay, where these kits can be easily purchased (Fig. 4.21).

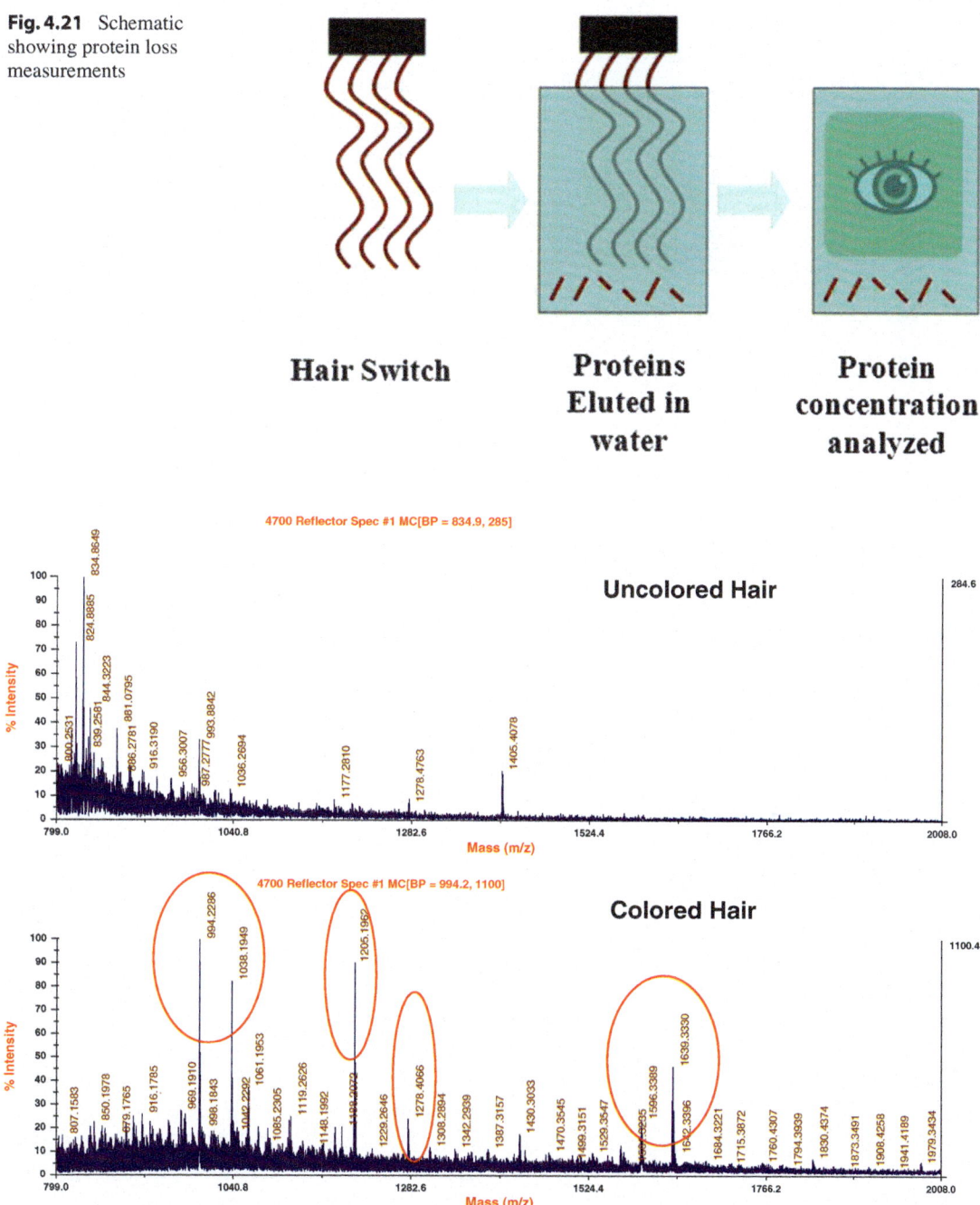

Fig. 4.21 Schematic showing protein loss measurements

Fig. 4.22 Mass spectroscopy data of soluble proteins diffusing out of hair that has not been coloured and hair after colouring

More sophisticated proteomic methods are available which involve identifying the precise protein fragments that are created during the damaging insult and which keratin protein they originate from. This is typically done using mass spectroscopy techniques and reference to databases where amino acid sequences for the majority of hair proteins can be identified. An example of this is the identification of protein fragments that are formed after treatment of hair with an oxidative colourant [2]. Figure 4.22 shows the mass spectra for the proteins diffused out of hair that is uncoloured and

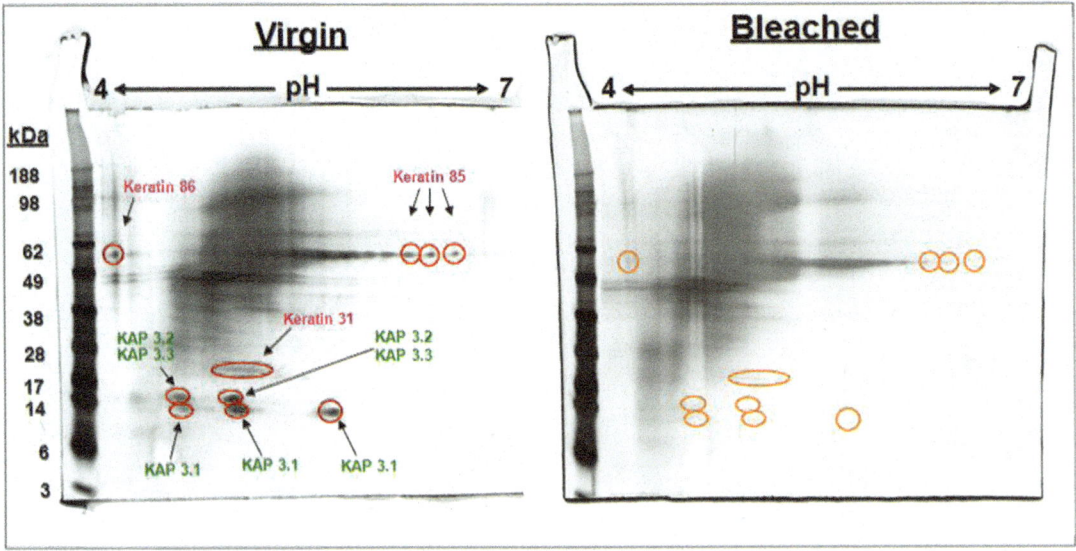

Fig. 4.23 2-D electrophoresis gels from virgin and bleached hair

coloured with the protein fragments formed by the colouring process highlighted. It has been shown that several of these soluble protein fragments are from keratin 31, a cortex-specific protein. Additional analysis on larger molecular weight fragments was sequenced as several type I (acidic) and type II (basic) keratin proteins. It is known these acidic and basic keratins associate together to form acid-base heterodimers and then heterodimers associate to from keratin filaments. Thus, with such proteomic techniques, it is possible to show specific locations of oxidative colourant damage in the cortex region of hair.

These methods measure proteins that diffuse out of hair, but proteomics may also be used to measure hair itself after exposure to a damaging insult.

2-D electrophoresis can separate hair proteins into different molecular weight and solubility families and then use mass spectroscopy methods to identify which proteins are changed. Figure 4.23 shows two 2-D gels from virgin and bleached hair where the proteins have been separated according to this method, and the image highlights areas where spots are present in the virgin sample but are missing in the bleached sample. Further analysis of the material in these highlighted areas can identify which proteins are missing in the bleached samples, and the figure illustrates locations of the keratin proteins and the keratin-associated proteins (KAPs). The data strongly suggests that bleaching can break down the protein structures in hair over multiple uses.

Summary

This section has outline some of the strategies and methodologies employed by the cosmetic researcher to relate the microscopic and macroscopic changes in the hair fibres and hair mass to what women see and feel in their regular lives. It further provides a basis to assess the performance of hair-care products designed to repair and protect hair health.

In the next chapter, we describe these products in some detail and offer practical advice in their use.

References

1. Reich C, Robbins C. Light scattering and shine measurements of human hair: a sensitive probe of the hair surface. J Soc Cosmet Chem. 1993;44:221–34.
2. Sinclair R, Flagler MJ, Jones L, Rufaut N, Davis MG. The proteomic profile of hair damage. Br J Dermatol. 2012;166 Suppl 2:27–32.

Clinical Signs of Hair Damage

Introduction

The environment causes daily damage to the hair shaft that cannot be repaired and is more evident in the distal part of long hair. Clinical signs of hair damage depend on type of damage and severity of damage. The resistance of hair to mechanical, physical, and chemical injuries is reduced in cases of hair diseases. Patients with hair disorders not only are more susceptible to hair damage because their hair is more delicate but often also utilise hairstyles that may cause or increase hair damage. Ethnicity is also important, as African hair is very easily damaged and broken by mechanical forces [1–3] and Asian hair is difficult to perm or dye due to its thick cuticle [4]. For these reasons, hair often becomes damaged after cosmetic procedures as it requires high concentrations of chemicals and long exposure.

Signs of hair damage include fragility, loss of lustre, dryness, and discoloration [5–7]. Damaged hair is non-appealing, as it looks dull, dry, and brittle. It is lighter than its original colour. It is difficult to style as it is frizzy and flyaway.

> **History**
> Trichorrhexis nodosa was first described by Samuel Wilks of Guy's Hospital in 1852, but M. Kaposi first coined this term in 1876 [8].

This chapter will discuss the clinical symptoms of hair damage, listed below, according to type of damage and ethnicity:

Symptoms of Hair Damage

- Hair breakage
- Hair tangling/matting
- Changes in the hair colour

> **Key Features**
> - Hair damage is more evident on the distal part of the hair shaft.
> - Patients with hair disorders are more susceptible to hair damage.
> - African hair is very easily damaged by mechanical, physical, and chemical insults.
> - Macroscopic signs of damage include fragility, loss of lustre, dryness, and discoloration.
> - Microscopic signs of hair damage include trichorrhexis nodosa, trichoclasis, trichoschisis, trichoptilosis, and bubble hair.
> - Symptoms include breakage, tangling, and matting.
> - Most common patient's complaint is slow or absent hair growth.

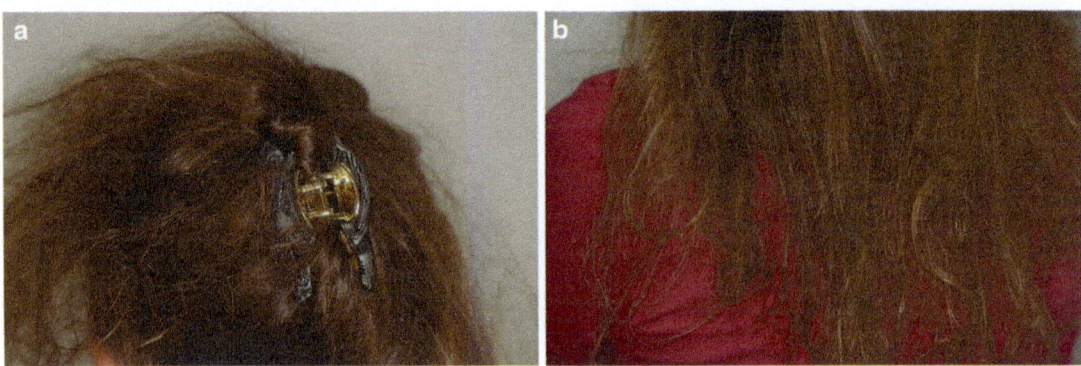

Fig. 5.1 This patient, affected by female pattern hair loss, (**a**) keeps her hair tightened with a clip to cover hair thinning. Note severe damage of the hair (**b**) which is dry, tangled, and with split ends

Hair Breakage

Severity of hair breakage depends on type of hair and type of damage. Patients may complain that their hair does not grow long or may consult because of patchy or diffuse alopecia. Diagnosis is confirmed by the 'tug' test and by the presence of trichorrhexis nodosa, which maybe often seen with the naked eye, but is more evident using dermoscopy or examining the hair under the microscope.

Other signs of hair weathering associated with breakage include trichoclasis, trichoschisis, trichoptilosis, and bubble hair [6, 7].

Causes

Causes of hair breakage include mechanical manipulation, friction, and exposure to excessive heat and chemical procedures [5]. Mechanical damage is most commonly due to brushing and combing. Different hair types react differently to combing forces, and African hair is more easily damaged, as its shape causes high friction between the hair fibres. Combing forces are lower for wet, curly hair versus dry, curly hair, as wetting the hair reduces the hair curvature, which also increases combing forces [9]. The opposite apply for straight Caucasian or Asian hair. Patchy alopecia due to trichorrhexis nodosa has been reported in young Indian men using a plastic comb to vigorously style their hair backwards 8–10 times a day [10].

Accessories used for styling such as hair clasps, pins, and rubber bands also can mechanically damage the hair and cause hair fracturing.

Friction due to the hairstyle is very common in women with androgenetic alopecia, who often wear their hair tightened back in a bun or in a ponytail to cover the thinning of the top of the scalp (Fig. 5.1a, b).

Excessive heat is very damaging for the hair, especially if utilised on wet hair or after applying a wet spray. Ceramic flat irons are often used daily and perceived as safe by consumers, even if they reach temperatures that are known to cause severe hair damage [11].

Chemical damage is more often caused by bleaching, perming, or straightening [12, 13]. Bleaching can leave the cuticles permanently raised and alter the moisture content of the hair shaft. Hair damage due to perming is caused either by over-perming or by incomplete neutralisation, most commonly due to shampoo in the hours following the procedure. Straightening is more risky than perming, as the hair is manipulated when its chemical bonds are broken.

Clinical Presentation

The clinical presentation depends on causes and ethnicity, as listed below. The most common hair shaft abnormalities include trichorrhexis nodosa, split ends, and fracture [14].

Introduction

Clinical Presentation Depending on Causes

- **Daily use of flat irons**: Trichorrhexis nodosa and breakage are more severe on the superficial upper hair shafts.
- **Excessive heat on wet hair**: Bubble hair.
- **Bleaching**: Hair is dull and dry, and trichorrhexis nodosa usually involves the tips.
- **Perming**: Localised or diffuse hair breakage is noted a few days after the procedure; breakage occurs a few centimetres from scalp emergency.
- **Straightening**: Breakage most commonly involves the nape area or the anterior scalp margin, where the chemical is first applied [2].

Clinical Presentation Depending on Ethnicity

- **African ancestry**: patchy or diffuse alopecia
- **Caucasians/Asians**: trichorrhexis nodosa, split ends

Trichorrhexis Nodosa

Trichorrhexis nodosa produces multiple white knots on the hair shaft, which corresponds to the sites of hair swelling and future fracturing (Fig. 5.2) [7, 8, 14].

Corresponding to these nodular swellings, the cuticle is lost and the exposed cortical fibres separate and fray (Fig. 5.3). At dermoscopy, the nodes appear as multiple white areas along the shafts (Fig. 5.4) [15]. These are more numerous on the shafts that have been lightened by chemical treatment or sunlight exposure (Fig. 5.5). The distal part, broken part of the shaft, has brush-like widened stump (Fig. 5.6).

Trichoptilosis

Trichoptilosis is the most common sign of weathering in long hair. The hair tips are frizzy and dry, and the distal ends of the hair shafts are

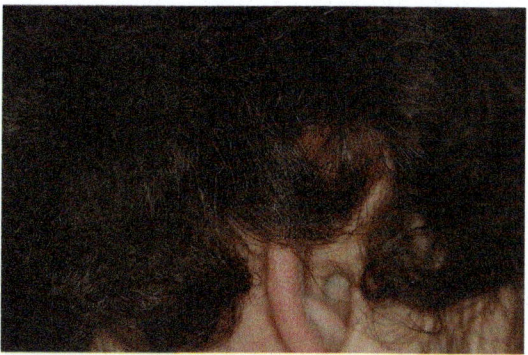

Fig. 5.2 Trichorrhexis nodosa: the hair of the parietal scalp shows multiple small, white spots

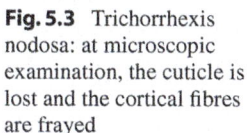

Fig. 5.3 Trichorrhexis nodosa: at microscopic examination, the cuticle is lost and the cortical fibres are frayed

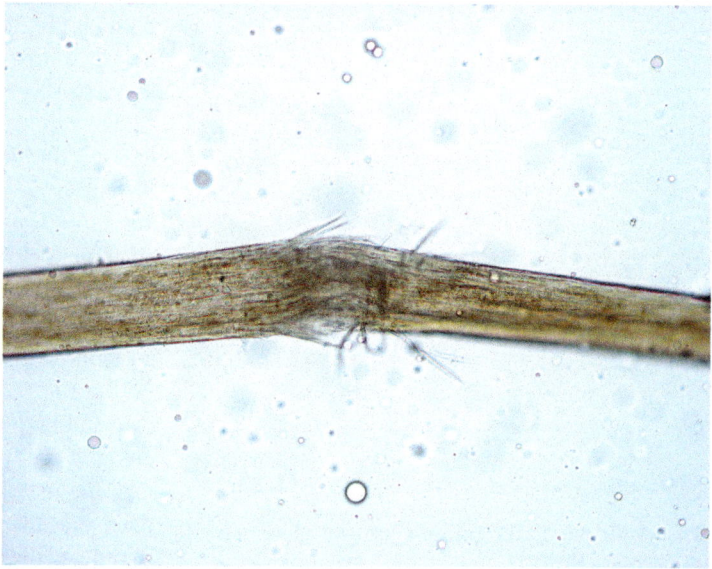

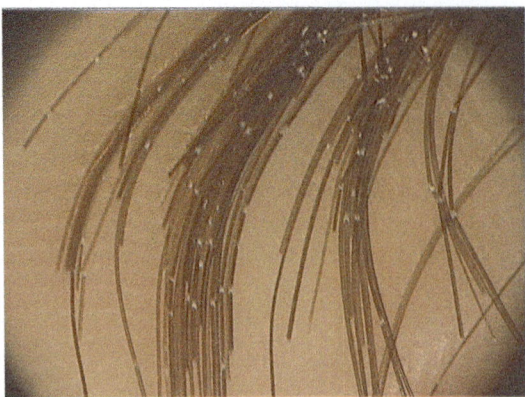

Fig. 5.4 Trichorrhexis nodosa: low-magnification dermoscopy showing multiple small, white swellings

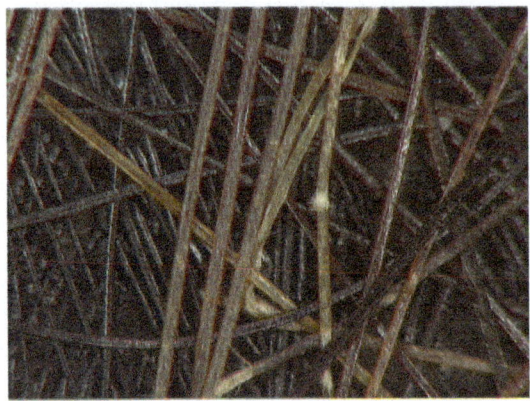

Fig. 5.5 Trichorrhexis nodosa: thrust paint brushes appearance at high magnification. Note selective involvement of lightened hairs

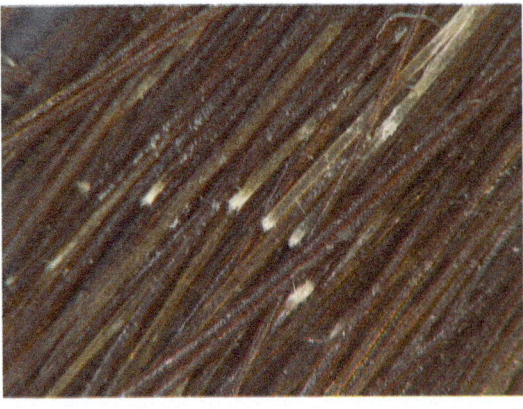

Fig. 5.6 Trichorrhexis nodosa: brush-like appearance of distal broken shafts

split longitudinally into two or several divisions (Fig. 5.7a, b) [16]. The bifurcated hair shaft is typically not surrounded by cuticle. Central trichoptilosis can also occur (Fig. 5.8); this is very common in African hair. Trichoptilosis is usually associated with other signs of hair damage, particularly trichorrhexis nodosa and trichonodosis.

Trichoschisis

The hair shaft shows a sharp transverse fracture, and breakage usually occurs at short distance from scarp emergency. This type of hair breakage is typically seen in trichothiodystrophy [17].

Trichoclasis

Trichoclasis is also a transverse fracture of the hair shaft, but different from trichoschisis, as the cuticle is not affected.

Bubble Hair

Bubble hairs are an uncommon sign of hair damage that can be due to excessive heat [18]. Patients are usually young females who use high heat, either in the form of blow dryers or electric curlers or, more commonly, straighteners, to style their hair [19]. Exposure of wet hair to excessive heat can cause sudden evaporation of water, with formation of cavities filled with steam within the hair shaft. At clinical examination, the hair breakage is usually more evident in the occipital and parietal region. Affected hair shows white, enlarged tips (Fig. 5.9a). At dermoscopy, the affected shaft has a spongy 'Swiss cheese' or 'honeycomb-like' appearance (Fig. 5.9b) [15], and microscopic examination reveals bubbles of different sizes that distend the hair shaft [20].

Alopecia due to Hair Breakage in Women of African Ancestry

Diffuse or patchy alopecia due to hair breakage is a common disease in women of African ancestry [2, 12, 21]. The African hair is, in fact, very delicate and highly susceptible to mechanical, physical, and chemical damage.

Patients present with diffuse (Fig. 5.10a) or patchy alopecia (Fig. 5.10b) and often do not correlate the hair problem with their styling

Introduction

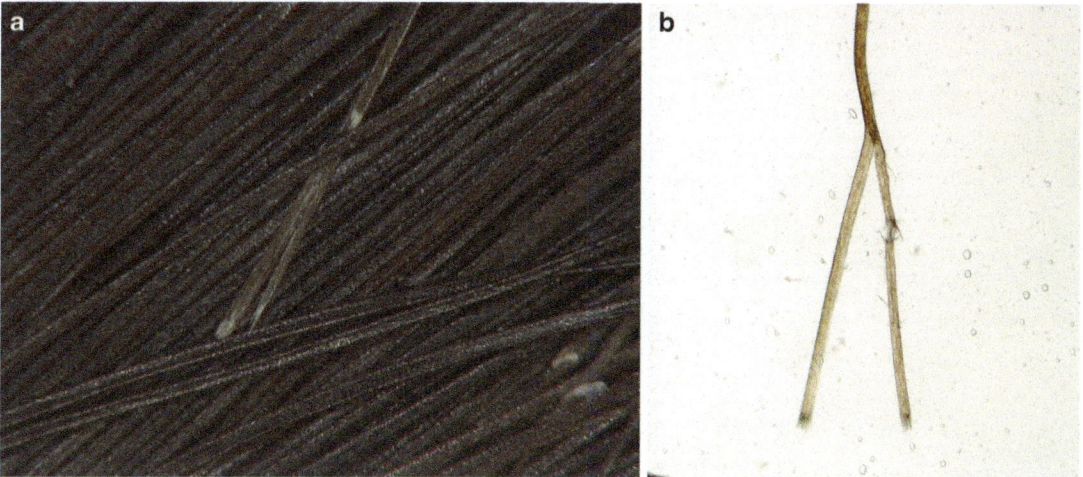

Fig. 5.7 Trichoptilosis: (**a**) dermoscopy shows hair shaft splitting and trichorrhexis nodosa. (**b**) Microscopic examination shows trichoptilosis and trichorrhexis nodosa

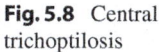

Fig. 5.8 Central trichoptilosis

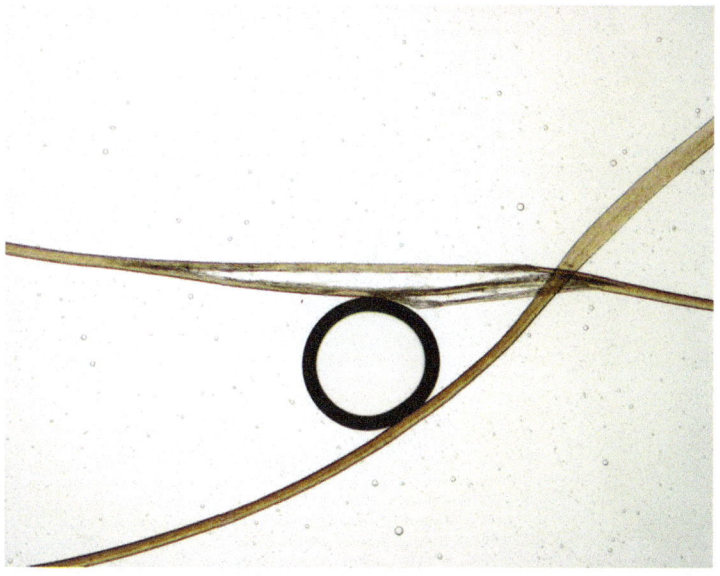

procedures. They usually complain of hair loss or that the hair does not grow.

Scalp dermoscopy of the alopecic scalp reveals a preserved honeycomb pattern and regularly distributed pinpoint white dots. The hair density in affected scalp areas is not reduced as compared with unaffected areas. Broken hairs maybe difficult to detect at dermoscopy as the hair is curly. However, hair fragments are usually present on clothes. Diagnosis is very easy and fast by observing with the microscope or the dermatoscope the hair fragments obtained with the tug test. These show longitudinal fissuring, knots, and brush-like ends due to trichorrhexis nodosa (Fig. 5.10c).

Hair Breakage in Caucasians and Asians

Caucasian and Asian patients usually complain that their hair is dull, dry, and flyaway and does not grow. Asian patients often complain that their

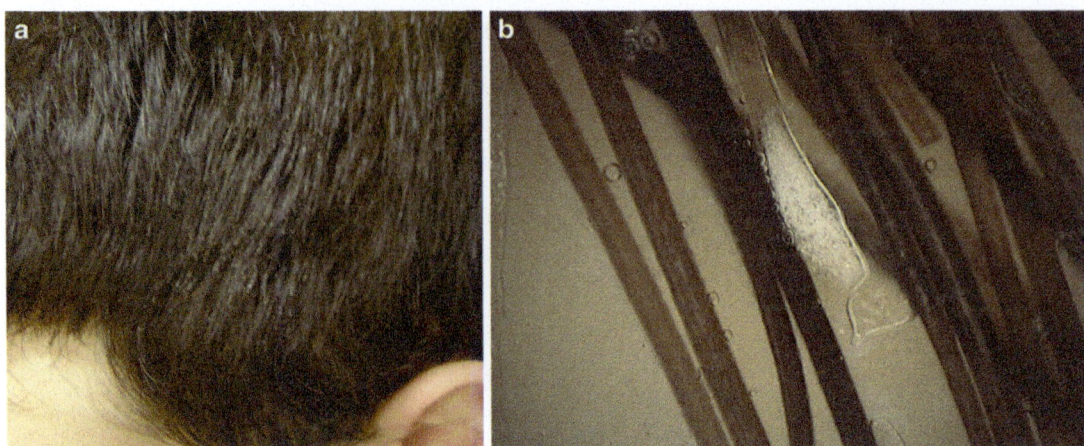

Fig. 5.9 Bubble hair: note (**a**) white, enlarged broken tips at clinical examination and (**b**) typical Swiss-cheese appearance at dermoscopy

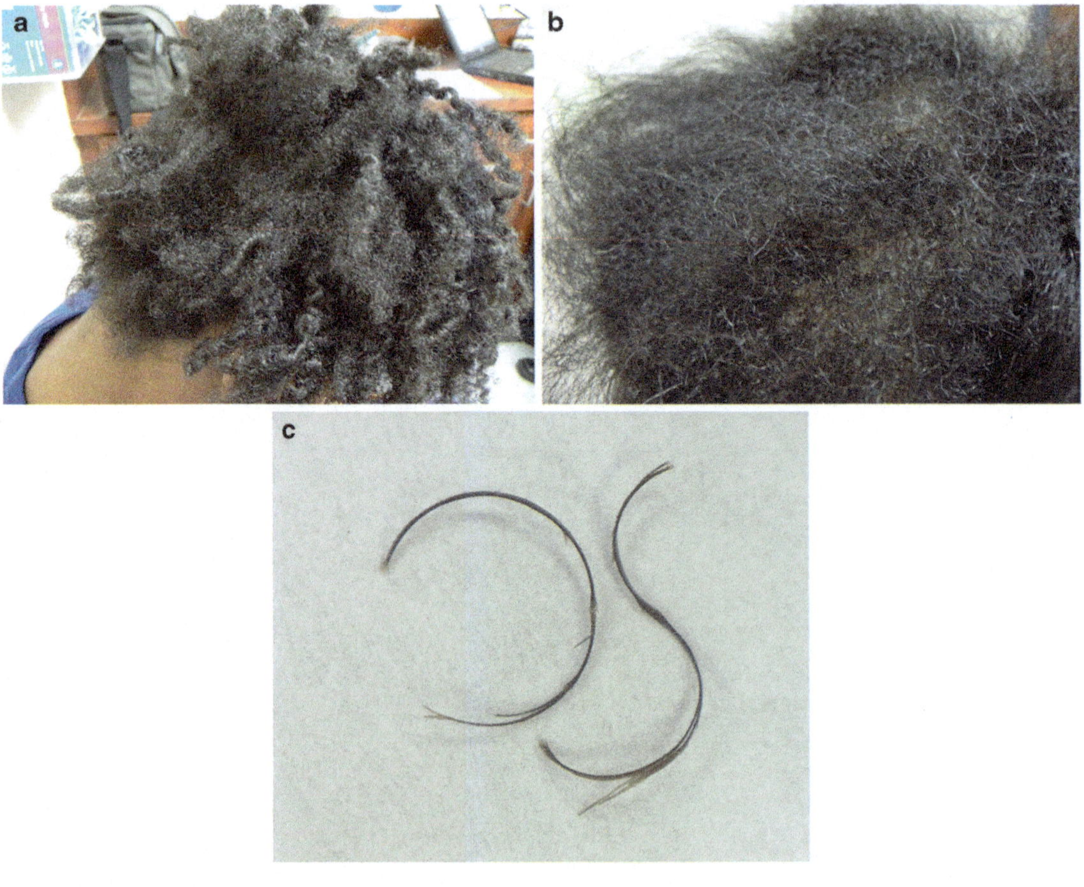

Fig. 5.10 (**a**) Diffuse or (**b**) patchy alopecia due to hair breakage in women of African ancestry. Diagnosis is easily confirmed by dermoscopy on the hair fragments obtained with the pull or the tug test: (**c**) note trichorrhexis and hair splitting

Introduction

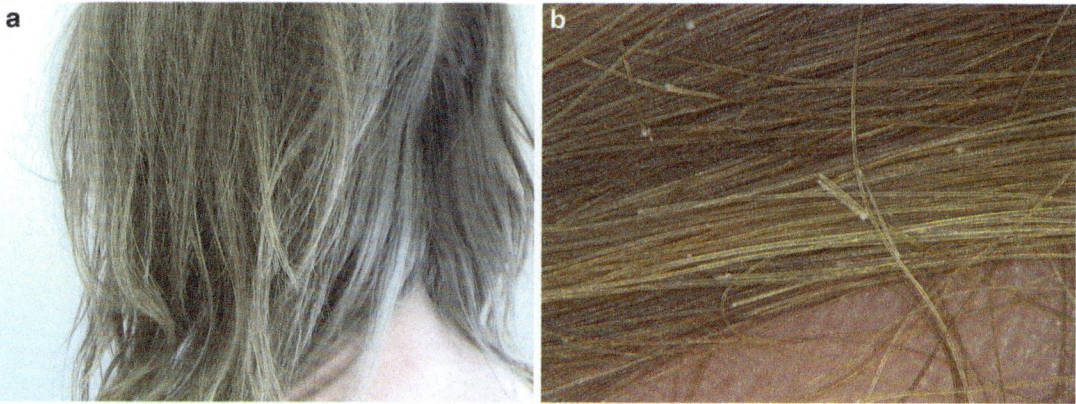

Fig. 5.11 The hair is (**a**) bleached and dry and shows signs of breakage and split ends; (**b**) dermoscopy confirms severe damage with trichorrhexis nodosa and breakage

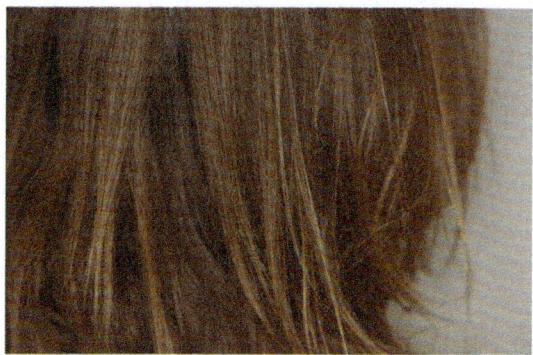

Fig. 5.12 Hair breakage causes blunt-ended hair of uneven lengths

hair is coarse and lacks softness. Patients usually do not link the hair problem to their styling procedures, but if asked, they admit chemical and thermal damage such as bleaching and straightening, often using a flat iron even daily. At clinical examination, the hair shows evident signs of chemical treatments (Fig. 5.11a, b). Breakage at different levels along the length of hair fibres causes broken blunt-ended hair of uneven lengths (Fig. 5.12). Damage is typically more severe on the superficial upper hairs, as the underlying hairs close to the scalp are usually not exposed to thermal damage, thus less or not affected at all. Careful examination reveals trichorrhexis nodosa and split ends (trichoptilosis). If asked, patients admit to finding small hair fragments in the basin after brushing or combing their hair.

Diagnosis

The tug test and dermoscopy allow a fast diagnosis of hair breakage. The cross-section trichometer can be useful to quantify severity of damage.

Tug Test

Diagnosis of hair breakage can easily be confirmed by the 'tug test' [22]. This can be done by holding with one hand a tuft of hair at 3–4 cm from their tips and tugging with the other hand the same tuft close to the tip. In this way, we cause mechanical breakage and obtain small fragments of hairs that can be examined under the microscope or with the dermatoscope.

Dermoscopy

The dermatoscope is very useful to detect trichorrhexis nodosa on the scalp and on the hair fragments [15]. At low magnification, the affected shafts show light-coloured nodules, which correspond to areas where the hair fibre structure is disrupted (see Fig. 5.4). At higher magnification, the areas of breakage resemble thrust paintbrushes, as they appear as the ends of two brushes aligned in opposition, as seen in Figs. 5.5 and 5.6.

Cross-Section Trichometer

This device measures the cross-sectional area of a bundle of hair and provides a numeric value, the hair mass index (HMI), that reflects thickness and density of the hairs in the selected bundle. When breakage is present, the bundle cross-sectional area decreases from the proximal portion toward the tip, and the ratio of the distal HMI to the proximal HMI can be used as an indicator of breakage severity [23].

Hair Knotting, Tangling, and Matting

Damaged hair is difficult to detangle and frequently develops localised matting. The causes and clinical presentation are discussed in this section.

Causes

Tangling and matting are due to friction and most commonly occur when the hair is wet. Hair matting has been assimilated to wool felting, where contiguous fibres compact under the influence of moisture, heat, and friction. In fact, wet hair has increased electrostatic forces and is more susceptible to the mechanical rotatory friction produced when shampooing. Tangling involves damaged shafts with trichorrhexis nodosa and raised cuticles. Rubbing wet hair after shampooing also favours tangling. Hair styles involving rubber bands and clasps also favour tangling and matting. Localised matting on the nape area is usually due to friction against pillows or sofas. Wearing extensions predispose to matting, as the telogen hairs that remain attached to the glued extensions easily tangle with the surrounding shafts.

Clinical Presentation

In hair knotting (trichonodosis), the hair shaft presents a single or double knot. The hair tends to splinter and fracture. The condition, which is more common in patients with curly hair, usually involves one or a few hair shafts and is caused by trauma due to friction, combing, brushing, and scratching. Hair knotting is very common in African hair.

Matting describes reversible or irreversible tangling of locks of hair, which stick together. Self-induced matting characterises the dreadlock

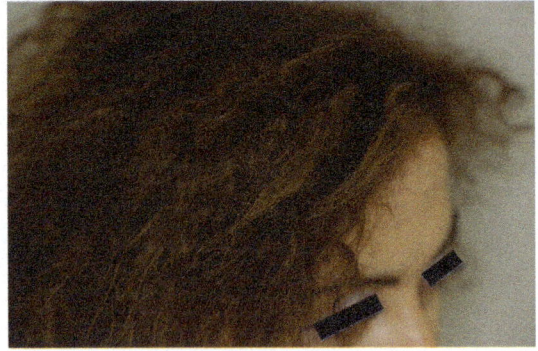

Fig. 5.13 Localised matting and breakage in a patient with severe hair weathering

hairstyle, where tufts of matted hair are on purpose kept long.

Localised matting is usually seen in Caucasian women with very damaged hair (Fig. 5.13). It is usually localised to the occipital hair, as friction plays an important role and may become first evident after prolonged bed rest (Fig. 5.14a, b). Although localised matting can be detangled with conditioning and gentle combing, it often tends to recur at the same site. A mild degree of irreversible tangling is common in individuals with long damaged hair and may require cutting of small hair tufts.

In patients wearing extensions, matting may involve any scalp area and is usually more evident 2 to 3 months of application of the extensions (Fig. 5.15a). The problem is more important in subjects with increased hair shedding. Clinical examination shows multiple white dots within the tangled area. These correspond to telogen roots entrapped by the glue at dermoscopy (Fig. 5.15b) [24].

Acute diffuse irreversible matting, reported as 'bird's-nest hair', is rarely observed in subjects with very damaged hair (Fig. 5.16a, b). The condition typically develops in patients with long hair who pile up the hair during shampooing, causing severe friction between the damaged hair fibres. Use of cationic surfactants has been implicated [25, 26]. Severe anagen effluvium has triggered acute matting in two patients with pancytopenia due to azathioprine. Possible precipitating factors include friction due to bed rest, hair shaft damage,

Introduction

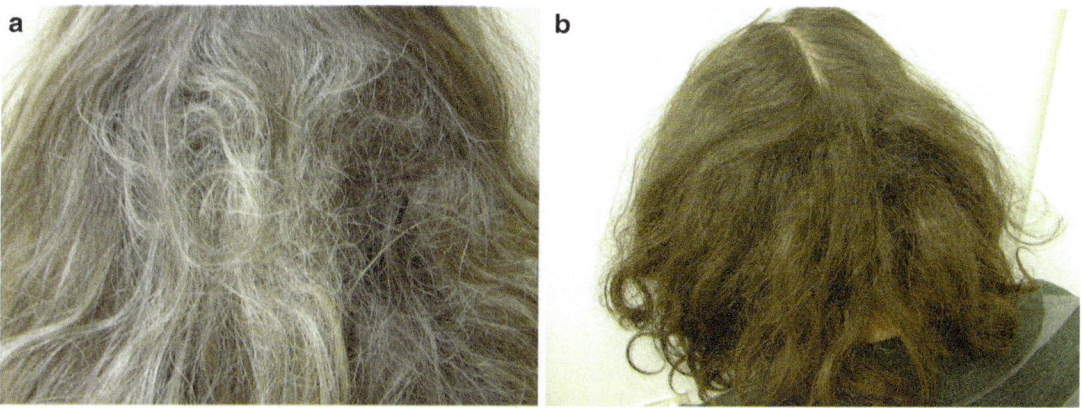

Fig. 5.14 (**a**, **b**) Localised matting in the occipital scalp favoured by friction

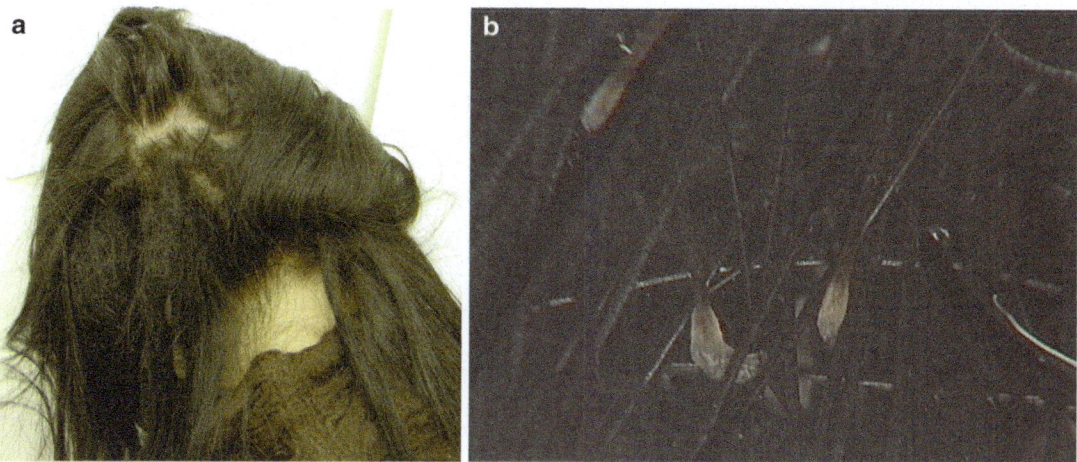

Fig. 5.15 (**a**) Localised matting in a patient wearing extensions. (**b**) Dermoscopy shows telogen roots entrapped in the matting

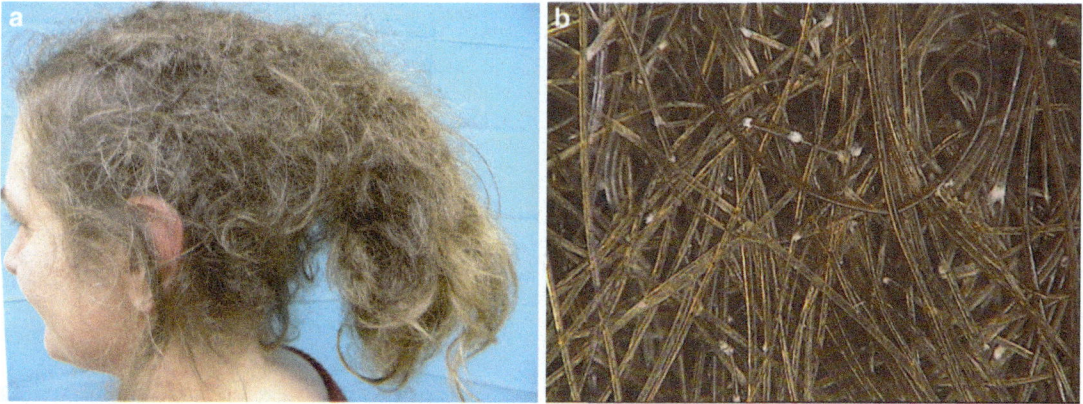

Fig. 5.16 (**a**) Acute irreversible matting in a patient with severe hair weathering. (**b**) Dermoscopy shows severe trichorrhexis nodosa

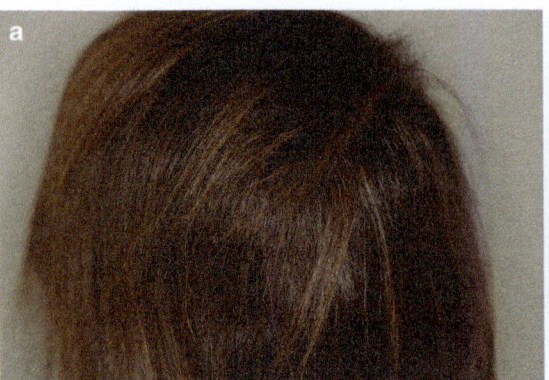
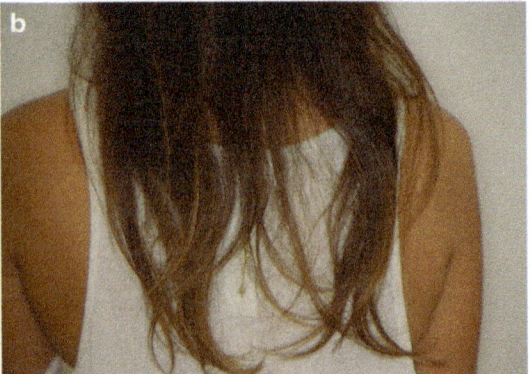

Fig. 5.17 Lightening of the (**a**) superficial exposed hair and (**b**) of the distal tips is a typical sign of hair damage

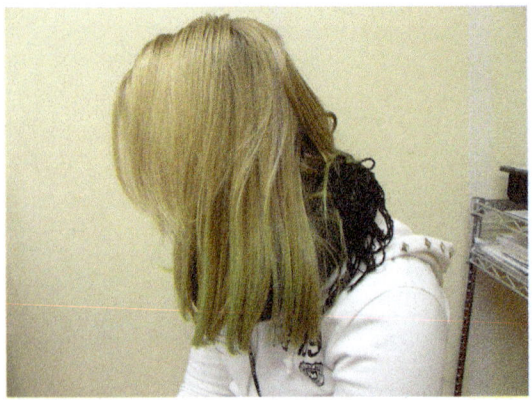

Fig. 5.18 Green hair in a patient with bleached, damaged hair

and hair shedding because of the medication with tangling of the shed shafts to the hair because patients were afraid of combing [27].

Changes in the Hair Colour

Exposed hair is bleached by sunlight [28]. Damaged hair is typically lighter in colour than the surrounding healthy hair. This is particularly evident in the tips of long hair. Dark hair lightens to a brownish-red colour; brown hair may become platinum blond (Fig. 5.17a, b).

Exposure to high concentrations of copper in tap water or swimming pools may cause green hair, particularly visible in blond subjects with damaged hair (Fig. 5.18) [29]. Green hair has also been reported after exposure to hair cosmetics [30, 31]. Possible treatments for green hair include use of shampoo containing a chelating agent or penicillamine.

Bleached hair may become reddish-brown after bathing in 'thermal' water or after use of topical medications.

References

1. Khumalo NP, Doe PT, Dawber RP, Ferguson DJ. What is normal black African hair? A light and scanning electron-microscopic study. J Am Acad Dermatol. 2000;43(5 Pt 1):814–20.
2. McMichael AJ. Hair breakage in normal and weathered hair: focus on the Black patient. J Investig Dermatol Symp Proc. 2007;12(2):6–9.
3. Franbourg A, Hallegot P, Baltenneck F, Toutain C, Leroy F. Current research on ethnic hair. J Am Acad Dermatol. 2003;48(6 Suppl):S115–9.
4. Takahashi T, Hayashi R, Okamoto M, Inoue S. Morphology and properties of Asian and Caucasian hair. J Cosmet Sci. 2006;4:327–38.
5. Dawber R. Cosmetic and medical causes of hair weathering. J Cosmet Dermatol. 2002;4:196–201.
6. Osorio F, Tosti A. Hair weathering, Part 1: Hair structure and pathogenesis. J Cosmet Dermatol. 2011;24: 533–8.
7. Osorio F, Tosti A. Hair weathering, Part 2: Clinical features, diagnosis, prevention and treatment. J Cosmet Dermatol. 2011;24:555–9.
8. Schwartz RA. Trichorrhexis nodosa. http://emedicine.medscape.com/article/1073664.
9. Robbins CR. Chemical and Physical Behavior of Human Hair. 5th ed. Berlin: Springer Verlag; 2012.
10. Martin AM, Sugathan P. Localised acquired trichorrhexis nodosa of the scalp hair induced by a specific

comb and combing habit – a report of three cases. Int J Trichol. 2011;3:34–7.
11. Mirmirani P, Christian P, Winsey N, Whatmough M, Cornwell PA. The effects of water on heat-styling damage. J Cosmet Sci. 2011;62:15–27.
12. Khumalo NP, Gumedze F. African hair length in a school population: a clue to disease pathogenesis? J Cosmet Dermatol. 2007;6:144–51.
13. Mamabolo T, Agyei NM, Summers B. Cosmetic and amino acid analysis of the effects of lye and no-lye relaxer treatment on adult black female South African hair. J Cosmet Sci. 2013;64:287–96.
14. Whiting DA. Structural abnormalities of the hair shaft. J Am Acad Dermatol. 1987;16:1–25.
15. Miteva M, Tosti A. Dermatoscopy of hair shaft disorders. J Am Acad Dermatol. 2013;68:473–81.
16. Lee HW, Choi JH, Moon KC, Koh JK. Trichoptilosis developing after first exposure to hair gels. Pediatr Dermatol. 2008;25:139–40.
17. Ferrando J, Mir-Bonafé JM, Cepeda-Valdés R, Domínguez A, Ocampo-Candiani J, García-Veigas J, et al. Further insights in trichothiodystrophy: a clinical, microscopic, and ultrastructural study of 20 cases and literature review. Int J Trichol. 2012;4:158–63.
18. Brown VM, Crounse RG, Abele DC. An unusual new hair shaft abnormality: "Bubble Hair". J Am Acad Dermatol. 1986;15:1113–7.
19. Detwiler SP, Carson JL, Woosley JT, Gambling TM, Briggaman RA. Bubble hair. Case caused by an overheating hair dryer and reproducibility in normal hair with heat. J Am Acad Dermatol. 1994;30:54–60.
20. Elston DM, Bergfeld WF, Whiting DA, McMahon JT, Dawson DM, Quint KL, et al. Bubble hair. J Cutan Pathol. 1992;19:439–44.
21. Rodney IJ, Onwudiwe OC, Callender VD, Halder RM. Hair and scalp disorders in ethnic populations. J Drugs Dermatol. 2013;12:420–7.
22. Mirmirani P, Huang KP, Price VH. A practical, algorithmic approach to diagnosing hair shaft disorders. Int J Dermatol. 2011;50:1–12.
23. Mhaskar S, Kalghatgi B, Chavan M, Rout S, Gode V. Hair breakage index: an alternative tool for damage assessment of human hair. J Cosmet Sci. 2011;62:203–7.
24. Yang A, Iorizzo M, Vincenzi C, Tosti A. Hair extensions: a concerning cause of hair disorders. Br J Dermatol. 2009;160:207–9.
25. Zawar VP, Mhaskar ST. Matting of hair following use of a new herbal shampoo. J Cosmet Dermatol. 2003;2:42–4.
26. Rigopoulos D, Kontochristopoulos G, Kalogirou O, Gregoriou S, Katsambas A. Matting of hair: what is the role of conditioners? J Eur Acad Dermatol Venereol. 2006;20:334–6.
27. Joshi R, Singh S. Plica neuropathica (plica polonica) following azathioprine-induced pancytopenia. Int J Trichol. 2010;2:110–2.
28. Santos Nogueira AC, Joekes I. Hair color changes and protein damage caused by ultraviolet radiation. J Photochem Photobiol B. 2004;74:109–17.
29. Fisher AA. Green hair: causes and management. Cutis. 1999;63:317–8.
30. Mascaró Jr JM, Ferrando J, Fontarnau R, Torras H, Domínguez A, Mascaró JM. Green hair. Cutis. 1995;56:37–40.
31. Tosti A, Mattioli D, Misciali C. Green hair caused by copper present in cosmetic plant extracts. Dermatologica. 1991;182:204–5.

Hair Density Reduction

Introduction

Hair loss is always very distressful and considerably impacts the patient's quality of life. Patients may complain of increased shedding, hair thinning, or both. It is therefore very important to assess both these parameters in all cases.

Increased hair shedding with almost normal hair density suggests telogen effluvium, which may be acute or chronic. A reduced hair density may involve the whole scalp (diffuse alopecia), may be limited to specific scalp regions (patterned alopecia), or may present with bald patches (patchy alopecia) [1, 2].

Acute Telogen Effluvium

Acute telogen effluvium results from conditions that induce the entry of a large number of hair follicles into their resting phase (telogen). Hair shedding is considered severe when more than 200 hairs are shed daily. Acute telogen effluvium develops 2–3 months after the triggering factor, and most common causes include systemic diseases, drugs, fever, stress, weight loss, delivery, iron deficiency, and inflammatory scalp disorders [3].

The patient usually remembers quite precisely when the increased shedding began. Acute telogen effluvium does not usually produce visible thinning, as up to 50 % of hairs need to be shed before reduction of hair density is evident.

Acute telogen effluvium can, however, unmask or worsen androgenetic alopecia, and it is always very important to exclude this diagnosis in patients complaining of increased hair shedding. Dermoscopy is very useful to detect initial androgenetic alopecia as a variability in the hair shaft diameter (Fig. 6.1) [4]. Recovery after acute telogen effluvium will affect the cosmetic appearance of the hair, as the patient will present many short hairs with a frizzy flyaway appearance. In the long term, hair will lose shine as alignment between the hair fibres is reduced.

Chronic Telogen Effluvium

Chronic telogen effluvium is not an acute telogen effluvium that prolongs for many months, but instead is a distinct condition that most commonly affects middle-aged women and frequently remains unexplained. Patients are usually very distressed and complain of progressive temporal thinning (Fig. 6.2) and decreased hair mass. They state that their ponytail is reduced to one third of the original mass. These patients often bring envelopes of shed hairs or pictures of the hair shed during shampoo (Fig. 6.3) to prove the amount of hair loss. At clinical exam, the hair density at scalp level looks normal or above the normal. Hair shedding is only slightly increased, and the pull test may be negative [5, 6]. Chronic telogen effluvium has a chronic course with periodic exacerbations.

Diffuse Alopecia

Anagen Effluvium

Anagen hair loss with diffuse alopecia is a typical side effect of cancer chemotherapy and scalp radiation. The alopecia is very severe and affects not only the scalp but also eyebrows, eyelashes, and body hairs. In most cases, complete regrowth is fast after discontinuation of therapy, but permanent alopecia may occur with high-dose radiation and certain drug regimens, such as busulfan and taxanes (Fig. 6.4) [7].

Patterned Alopecia (Androgenetic Alopecia)

Androgenetic alopecia, which is the most common form of hair loss, affects up to 80 % of men (male pattern hair loss) and 50 % of women (female pattern hair loss) in the course of their life. Androgenetic alopecia is caused by a reduction in the thickness, length, and pigmentation of the hair. In males, hair thinning is limited to the frontotemporal areas and the vertex. In women, the condition produces a diffuse thinning of the crown region with maintenance of the frontal hairline. This pattern is better appreciated by making a central parting and comparing hair density at the top with hair density at the occipital region [8, 9].

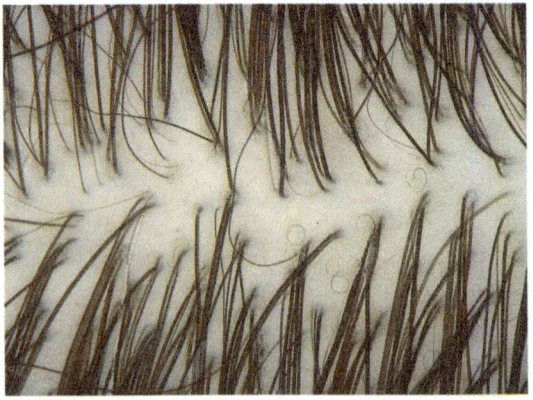

Fig. 6.1 Dermoscopy shows hair shafts of different thickness. Variability affects more than 20 % of the shafts; this is diagnostic for androgenetic alopecia

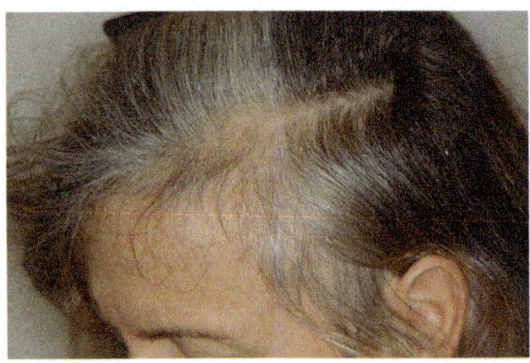

Fig. 6.2 Chronic telogen effluvium: note thinning of the temporal region

Fig. 6.3 Patients often bring pictures of the hairs shed during shampoo to prove the hair loss

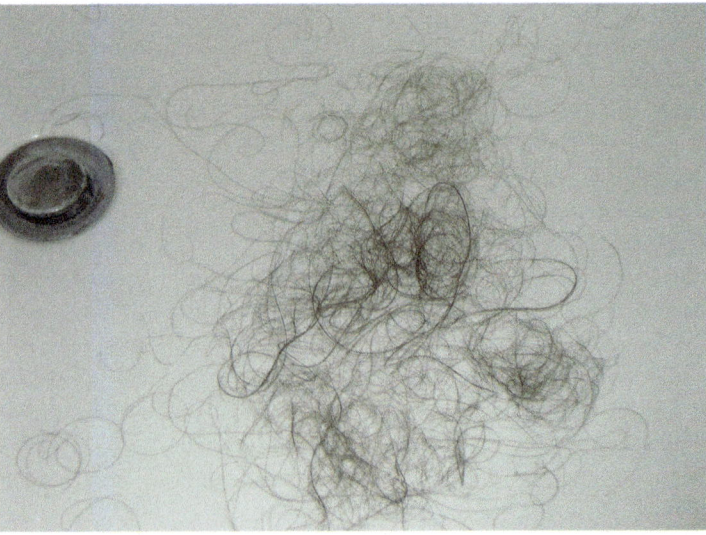

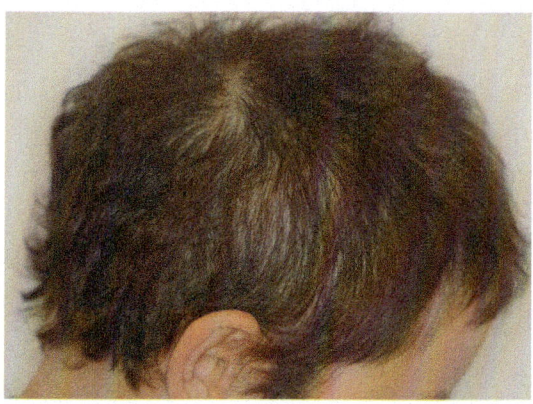

Fig. 6.4 Permanent alopecia after chemotherapy. Hair density and length are considerably reduced

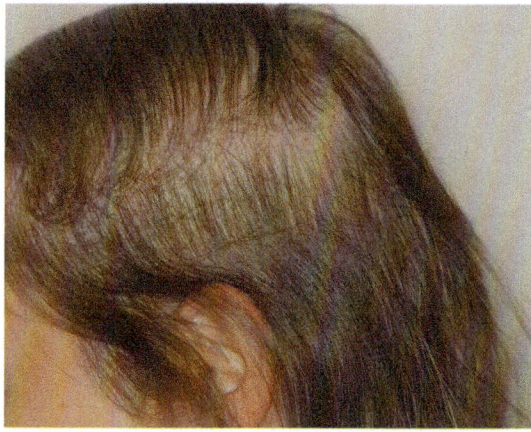

Fig. 6.5 Androgenetic alopecia: hair thinning often affects parietal and occipital areas

Some women may present a very diffuse thinning involving the parietal and occipital scalp (Fig. 6.5). Hair thinning is commonly associated with hair shaft damage. The hair mass is greatly reduced, and patients present sparse, uneven ends.

Alopecia Areata

Alopecia areata is a common form of nonscarring, usually patchy, hair loss affecting up to 2 % of the population. Clinical examination reveals one or multiple well-circumscribed smooth patches of alopecia that enlarge in a centrifugal way. Severe forms involve the entire scalp (alopecia totalis) or all body hair (alopecia universalis) [10].

References

1. Tosti A, Piraccini BM, Sisti A, Duque-Estrada B. Hair loss in women. Minerva Ginecol. 2009;61(5):445–52.
2. Shapiro J. Hair loss in women. N Engl J Med. 2007;357(16):1620–30.
3. Headington JT. Telogen effluvium: new concepts and review. Arch Dermatol. 1993;129:356–63.
4. Miteva M, Tosti A. Hair and scalp dermatoscopy. J Am Acad Dermatol. 2012;67(5):1040–8.
5. Whiting DA. Chronic telogen effluvium: increased scalp hair shedding in middle-aged women. J Am Acad Dermatol. 1996;35(6):899–906.
6. Gilmore S, Sinclair R. Chronic telogen effluvium is due to a reduction in the variance of anagen duration. Australas J Dermatol. 2010;51(3):163–7.
7. Palamaras I, Misciali C, Vincenzi C, Robles WS, Tosti A. Permanent chemotherapy-induced alopecia: a review. J Am Acad Dermatol. 2011;64(3):604–6.
8. Blume-Peytavi U, Blumeyer A, Tosti A, Finner A, Marmol V, Trakatelli M, et al. S1 guideline for diagnostic evaluation in androgenetic alopecia in men, women and adolescents. Br J Dermatol. 2011;164(1):5–15.
9. Herskovitz I, Tosti A. Female pattern hair loss. Int J Endocrinol Metab. 2013;11(4), e9860.
10. Alkhalifah A, Alsantali A, Wang E, McElwee KJ, Shapiro J. Alopecia areata update: Part I. Clinical picture, histopathology, and pathogenesis. J Am Acad Dermatol. 2010;62(2):177–88.

Cosmetic Products and Hair Health

Introduction

In previous chapters we explored the sequence of events which renders a healthy head of hair 'unhealthy'. Disruption of the normal structure and physiology of the hair shafts renders them dry and weak, and ultimately leads to an unmanageable head of hair lacking shine and prone to breakage and/or frizz (Fig. 7.1a–d).

Although it is neither possible to 'cure' the chemical disruption of repeated bleaching nor to permanently mend split ends, it is possible to mitigate these changes with sensible hair-care practices and regular use of high-quality hair-care products. As with most disorders, prevention is better than cure.

Selection of the correct products from the plethora facing women in the stores is not necessarily intuitive. The desire for constant change, which is a hallmark of the age, leads to constantly changing to different product ranges. Research demonstrates that this offers no advantage and, indeed, is potentially deleterious. A clear understanding of the state of the hair, selection of the correct regimen type to address this, and the regular use of these products is the key to prolonged hair health.

In this chapter, the science of hair-care products is allied to a practical guide on the selection of the correct regimen based on hair type. A graphic illustration using examples from an expert stylist and the home situation reveals how the application of high-quality hair-care products and sensible hair-care practices can improve hair health.

The History of Hair Care and Hair-Care Products

The desire for personal cleanliness is recorded in the earliest Mediterranean civilisations more than 3000 years ago. It perpetuated through the Roman and the Byzantine empires, where guaranteed water supplies established both private and public baths and even showers. Soaps made from animal fats boiled with ashes have been found in archaeological excavations, but it can be imagined that mildness and cleansing efficacy were not major attributes. Hair was often dressed with oils as an alternative strategy.

In the Middle Ages, public bathing was common, although this fell away until the twentieth century when domestic water supplies became commonplace. In Japan and Mesoamerica, bathing was prized, and in the seventeenth century, there was a mention of hair washing but without detailing products. It is the guaranteed supply of water which is critical to bathing and particularly hair washing. Even today in parts of Africa

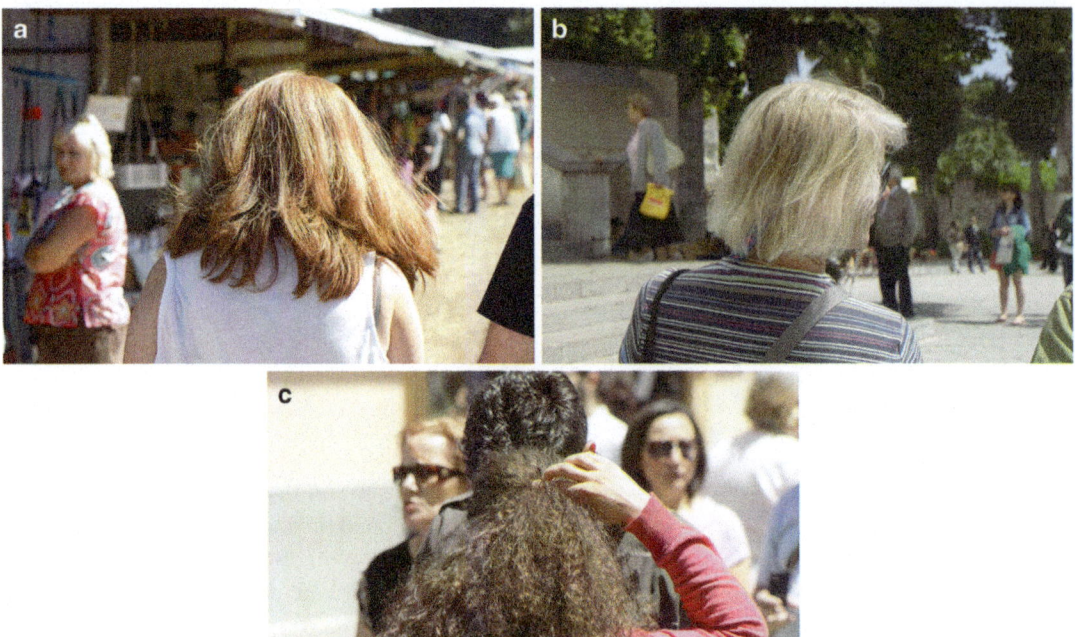

Fig. 7.1 (**a–c**) Disruption of the normal structure and physiology of the hair shafts results in dry, weak, and unmanageable heads of hair lacking shine

bathing, and especially shampooing, is as low as 20th on the list of priorities for such a precious resource.

Shampoo (derived from the Hindustani word *champo-*) appeared in Europe from China and is first recorded in English in 1762 as a head massage consisting of alkalis, oils, and fragrances. Shaved soap was boiled in water and herbs were added; this mixture was meant to give the hair shine and fragrance and was presumably considered 'leading-edge technology' of the day. Of the plethora of homemade products, ingredients such as beer, lemon juice, and eggs have been used to give shine—an attribute, as we have seen, that is key to denoting healthy hair.

Shampoos are the bedrock of hair care, cleansing the hair and preparing it for conditioning and styling. The first synthetic (non-soap) shampoo *Drene* was introduced in the 1930s. Products have since evolved dramatically and not only gently cleanse hair but, correctly applied, are also able to protect its structure and enhance its aesthetics. Other than 'clarifying' shampoos, conditioning actives are now discretely delivered to hair from most quality shampoos.

Conditioners were developed as an adjunct to shampoos to control the flux of moisture in and out of the hair fibre, provide lubrication to minimise friction-related damage, reduce static charge, and smooth rough surfaces. Their contribution to feel, appearance, resilience, manageability, and overall hair health has been significant. However, on a global basis, conditioning still falls far below the frequency of shampooing.

In recent decades, hair-care products have been transformed from the functional, but often mildly unpleasant, to versatile, creative, and quality-of-life enhancing. Conditioners are now available as regular rinse-out, leave-in, lightweight, or intensive variants and are designed to

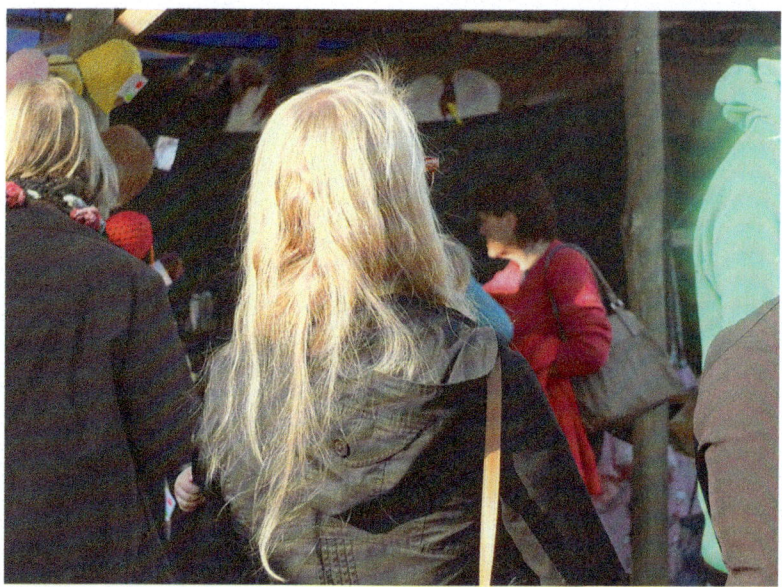

Fig. 7.2 Research indicates that, overall, hair health is worse now than a decade ago

meet a range of challenges in hair health. In an increasingly competitive society of the twenty-first century, the prolonged wearing of unwashed and matted hair might be considered eccentric at the very least and antisocial at worst. Sadly, from the recent research (P&G data on file), the level of hair health is measurably worse than a decade ago, despite hair-care products being more innovative and effective (Fig. 7.2a–c).

To restore hair health, a hair-care REGIMEN is necessary. This is a combination of products selected for an individual's hair type and desired end benefit and which fits with their lifestyle and economic circumstance.

Hair-Care Regimens

A basic hair-care regimen includes a shampoo, a range of conditioning variants, and ancillary products such as serums, heat protectors, smoothing agents, and styling products.

History of Regimens for Different Hair Types

Regimen ranges were once designed for perceived hair 'types' differences. Products labelled for *normal*, *dry*, *oily*, or *damaged* hair abounded on supermarket shelves. In response to women's feedback, subsequent formulations were created to deliver what is termed 'desired end benefit' of which 'smooth and sleek', 'perfect curls', and 'colour radiant' are examples.

At the same time, a parallel 'ethnic' business developed products designed for dry and tightly curled hair and based on the essential need for moisturisation. These products are often formulated with more intensive conditioning agents, like petrolatum, and contain product forms such as pomades, which can have a greasy and waxy consistency. Unlike hair spray and hair gel, pomades do not dry and often takes several washes to remove.

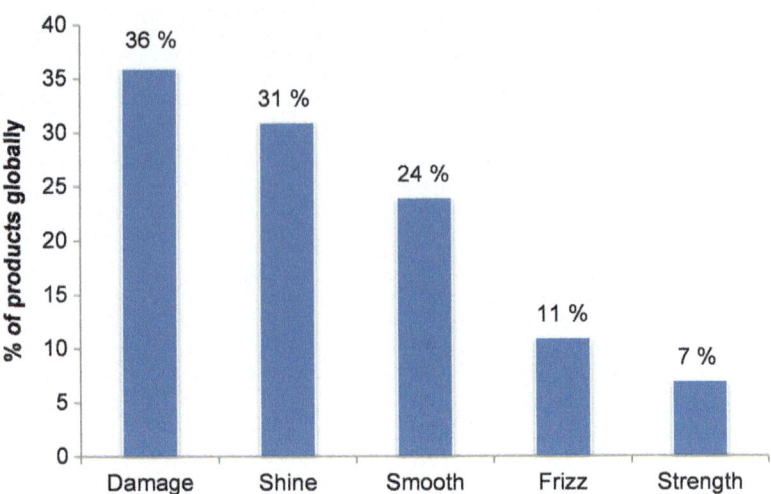

Fig. 7.3 Percentage of products which refer to aspects of hair health in their product description

Product Development for Hair Health

The hair-care industry has developed many different technology options and formulations to address women's needs in the area of hair health. The retail hair-care industry is predicted to be worth approximately $60 billion by 2016. A significant portion of products are targeted either directly to hair health and damage or specifically to the key signals of hair health such as shine, strength, and frizz.

In 2013, approximately 11,000 new products were launched globally across the four major categories—shampoos, conditioners, styling products, and treatments (data from Mintel Global New Products Database). Despite this large number of products, there are a set of common benefits driven mainly by women's hair needs. The top needs are as follows: volume, cleaning, controlling curls, smoothness, moisture renewal, anti-breakage, shine, protecting against colour fade, and repair and protection from damage. Some of these benefits are targeted at end look and feel benefits related to hair health such as volume, shine, and moisture renewal, and some are related to prevention and repair of damage. Out of the 11,000 products, 35 % contain reference to the product targeting hair damage, 31 % targeting hair shine, and 24 % targeting hair smoothness. These hair health benefits are fairly evenly distributed across product forms. An exception is treatments which are more focused on damage repair and prevention (Fig. 7.3).

Hair Health Connections

In the latest hair-care products, there are many different technologies which are either targeted to a damage insult or targeted specifically to achieving the final benefit. In some instances, the same material will drive a number of different end points. The schematic below shows some of these connections (Fig. 7.4). This schematic demonstrates that conditioning ingredients such as silicones, quats, fatty alcohols, and polymers contribute a significant percentage of protection for different sources of damage and drive an equally significant percentage of signals of hair health.

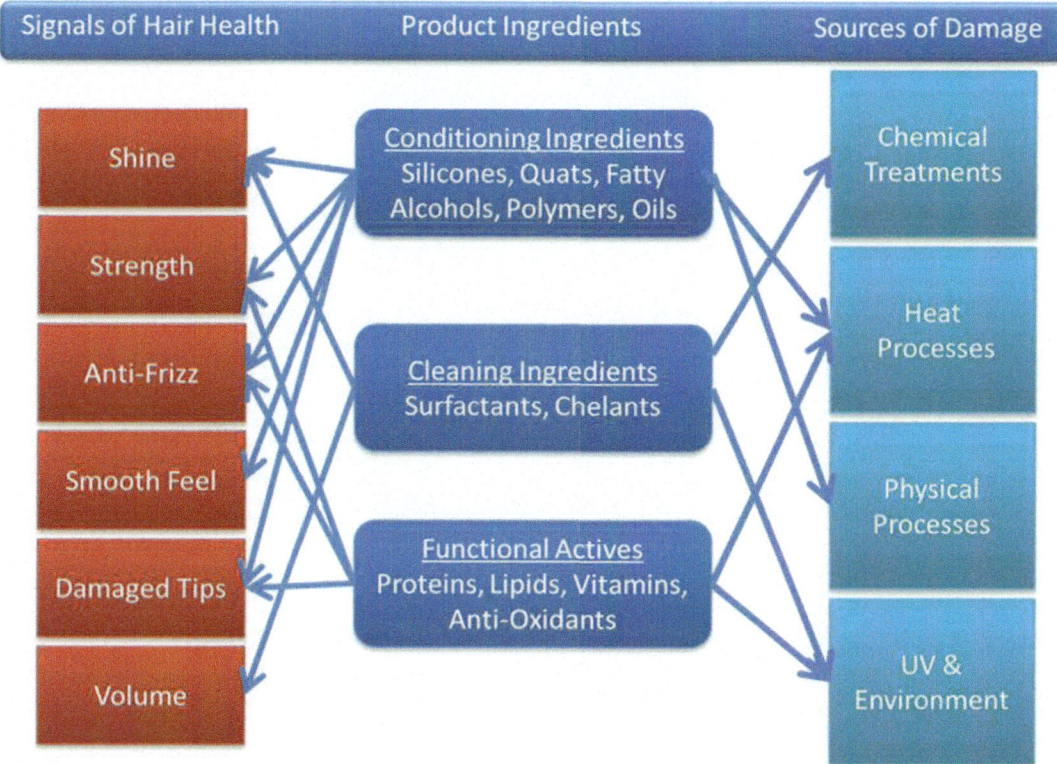

Fig. 7.4 Hair health connections

Hair-Care Products for Different Hair Needs

There are factors which the cosmetic industry takes into account when designing a regimen for different needs and which, to a large measure, are independent of regional stereotypes, although in areas such as the Americas and increasingly in Europe, all phenotypes are present in the marketplace. Product ranges are now designed to manage fine, thick, curly, and chemically damaged hair wherever they occur.

In this section, we examine the specific ingredients which are incorporated in the leading hair-care products and which are essential for the maintenance or restoration of hair health.

Shampoos

Early products were relatively inefficient, and many were harsh to the cuticular surface, the skin, and the eyes. Today, such products are highly efficient, aesthetically pleasing, and mild to those surfaces they touch. In addition to removing sebum from the hair and the detritus it inevitably collects, many shampoos now contain ingredients that are designed to enhance the natural properties of hair and mitigate environmental and self-inflicted damage. Products carry ingredient labels in compliance with worldwide and company regulations (Fig. 7.5) Hair-care products, in comparison to skin care products, are inexpensive and widely distributed.

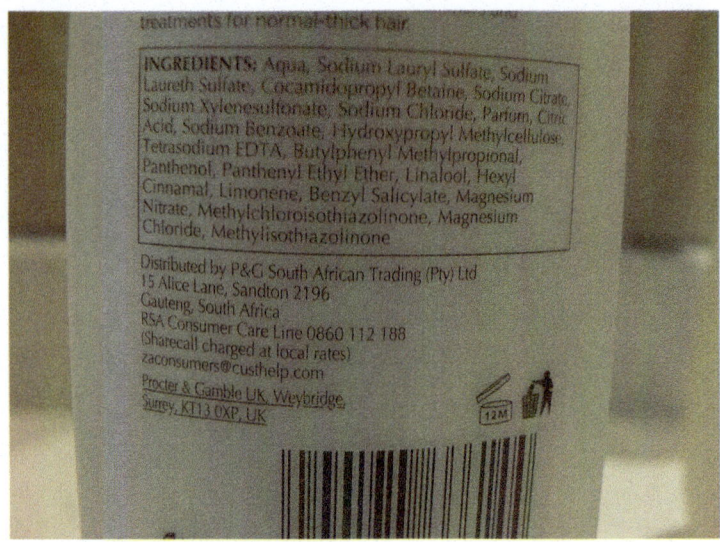

Fig. 7.5 Products carry ingredient labels in compliance with worldwide and company regulations

General Attributes of Shampoos

Shampoo formulations seek to maximise the following qualities:

- Effective cleaning
- Easy rinsing
- Good finish after washing hair
- Pleasant in-use aesthetics (lather, product thickness, perfume, etc.)
- Minimal skin/eye irritation
- No damage to hair
- Outstanding safety profile
- Good biodegradability

Modern Shampoo Formulations

Shampoos are invariably an aqueous (water-based) product and consist of three major components:

1. Primary surfactants for removing dirt and providing foaming power
2. Secondary surfactants to improve and condition the hair
3. Additives which complete the formulation and add special aesthetic effects and endow secondary benefits such as volume and shine

Surfactant Mode of Action

Both soaps and shampoos contain surfactants—compounds that lower the surface tension between a liquid and a solid. They may act as detergents (a mixture of surfactants with cleaning properties in dilute solutions), wetting agents, emulsifiers, foaming agents, or dispersants.

Soaps can bind to oils with such affinity that they remove too much if used on hair. Shampoos use certain surfactants balanced to provide the level of surface cleaning suited to hair fibres. These surfactant systems are called **syndets**—synthetic/detergents which are manufactured with a range of properties.

Undamaged hair has a negatively charged hydrophobic (water-resistant) surface to which lipids (fats) adhere, but from which water is initially repelled. Sebum and detritus are not easily removed when the hair is rinsed with plain water. Shampoo applied to wet hair is absorbed into the oil/hair interfaces.

A surfactant inherently moves toward 'surfaces' and cleans hair by removing dirt and oils (sebum) that are not water soluble. It also forms a lather, which is a signal desired by many to show that the shampoo is working.

A surfactant has a head group that is hydrophilic (water loving/oil hating) and a tail group that is hydrophobic (water hating/oil loving).

Surfactants will either migrate to the air/water interface or to an oil material with their hydrophilic head group toward the water and the hydrophobic tail group toward the oil or air. The surfactant will try to surround the oil droplet and, in doing so, will lift it off the surface where it will be rinsed off down the drain.

The three types of surfactants or detergents found in shampoos are:

- Anionic
- Nonionic
- Amphoteric

Anionic
These have a negatively charged hydrophilic component and are mainly used as primary surfactants. Laureth sulphates and lauryl sulphates are often used to gently cleanse. They are highly effective and possess the foaming properties that are desired by women. Products which do not foam are often regarded as 'ineffective' and may reduce compliance.

Nonionic
These surfactants condition the hair and perform gentle cleansing. They can increase the quality of lather in a shampoo, as well as its viscosity and solubility. They can be added for mildness or to improve the anti-static qualities of a shampoo, e.g. ethoxylated fatty alcohols.

Amphoteric
These surfactants contain a balance of positive and negative charges. They are very mild cleansers. They condition the hair but are generally less effective cleaners than anionic surfactants. They are also nonirritating to the eyes, which is why they are commonly used in baby shampoos.

Key Ingredients of Shampoos

In Table 7.1, the key ingredients of shampoos are described and the chemical names found on products are included.

Controversies

Sulphates
Shampoo products contain surfactants whose main purpose is to clean hair of sebum lipids and also dirt, dust, and skin flakes that collect on hair during the day. There has been considerable debate in the literature and media whether the class of surfactants called sulphates are detrimental to the hair and inherently to hair health. Products are labelled 'sulphate-free' with the imputation that sulphate-containing formulations

Table 7.1 Key ingredients of shampoos

Material class	Name to look for on products	Function
Surfactant	Sodium lauryl sulphate, sodium laureth sulphate, cocamidopropyl betaine	Cleans sebum, dust, and dirt from hair as well as previously applied product (e.g. gels, hairsprays) Provides lather
Silicone	Dimethicone	Makes hair easier to comb, softer, and smoother Increases shine by increasing fibre to fibre alignment
Polymer	Polyquaternium-76, guar hydroxypropyltrimonium chloride, polyquaternium-6, hydroxypropyl methylcellulose	Provides wet feel Aids in depositing silicone conditioning materials on hair
Additional ingredients	Panthenol, vitamin E, trisodium ethylenediamine disuccinate	Targeted benefits, e.g. moisturisation, antioxidant, chelant for UV protection

are inherently harsh or damaging. However, sulphate-free does not mean surfactant-free. The chemistry of a shampoo focuses on activity on the surface to remove sebum and detritus, not by ingredients working individually or penetrating the surface to 'strip' the cuticle.

A shampoo is a complex but essentially aqueous solution with key ingredients in relatively low concentrations. Mildness (or otherwise) is the function of how surfactants are balanced within the total formulation, not whether any specific and isolated ingredient is more aggressive than others. Shampoos with alternative surfactants which might be intrinsically labelled mild are frequently less effective. Fortunately, women select on whether a product works, is aesthetically pleasing, and is cost effective.

Specialised Shampoos

Antidandruff

In addition to regular shampoos, the most popular scalp products sold worldwide are targeted at preventing dandruff, a condition which affects over half the adult population at some time in their lives. Actives such as zinc pyrithione, climbazole, and salicylic acid are used in both shampoos and conditioners to improve scalp health by the elimination of the putative fungus *Malassezia globosa* and reduce surface sebum levels. If used regularly, they can prevent signs and symptoms of dandruff.

Conditioning (2-in-1) Shampoos

Combination, or 2-in-1, products were developed first by Procter and Gamble in the late 1980s and delivered for the first time cleansing and conditioning benefits from a single product source. Since this innovation, it has become possible and commonplace to incorporate conditioning ingredients into shampoos—primarily to prevent tangling, but also to facilitate styling.

The challenge was to deliver conditioning actives from a product that has to both clean hair and deposit conditioning ingredients onto the hair surface. The main mechanism of achieving this is via a coacervate formation wherein an anionic polymer is formulated with a surfactant and silicone to deposit the silicone on hair as the shampoo is diluted during rinsing (Figs. 7.6a, b and 7.7a, b).

There exists a range of polymers that can be used for this, including natural polymers, celluloses, and synthetic polymers. These play a role in creating the coacervate (a miniscule spherical droplet of assorted molecules which is held together by hydrophobic forces from a surrounding liquid). This enables deposition of silicone on hair, but in some cases, they can imbue wet feel benefits. Consequently, hair can feel smooth during shampooing and with decreased friction forces.

'Natural' Shampoos

Some products claim to include 'all-natural', 'organic', or 'botanical' ingredients (such as plant extracts). The effectiveness of these organic ingredients alone can be controversial. Other products contain organic or botanicals in addition to a standard surfactant system.

Shampoos for Children

Shampoo for infants is formulated so that it is the same pH level as the eye, making it less irritating if it were to get into the eyes. Most contain sodium laureth sulphate and/or sodium lauryl sulphate. Alternatively, infant shampoos may be formulated using other classes of surfactants, most notably nonionics which are much milder than any charged anionics used.

Moisturising Shampoos

Moisturising products fill a huge need both globally and across all hair types. Moisturisation is not the same as adding moisture to hair and is more about delivering a soft and conditioned feel. In fact, it has been shown that hair with higher moisture actually feels drier than hair with low moisture levels. The benefit can be delivered at different levels depending on the product. There are very intense formulations for women with very damaged and dry hair and lightweight versions for women who want conditioned feel but are concerned about a trade-off of having hair weighed down.

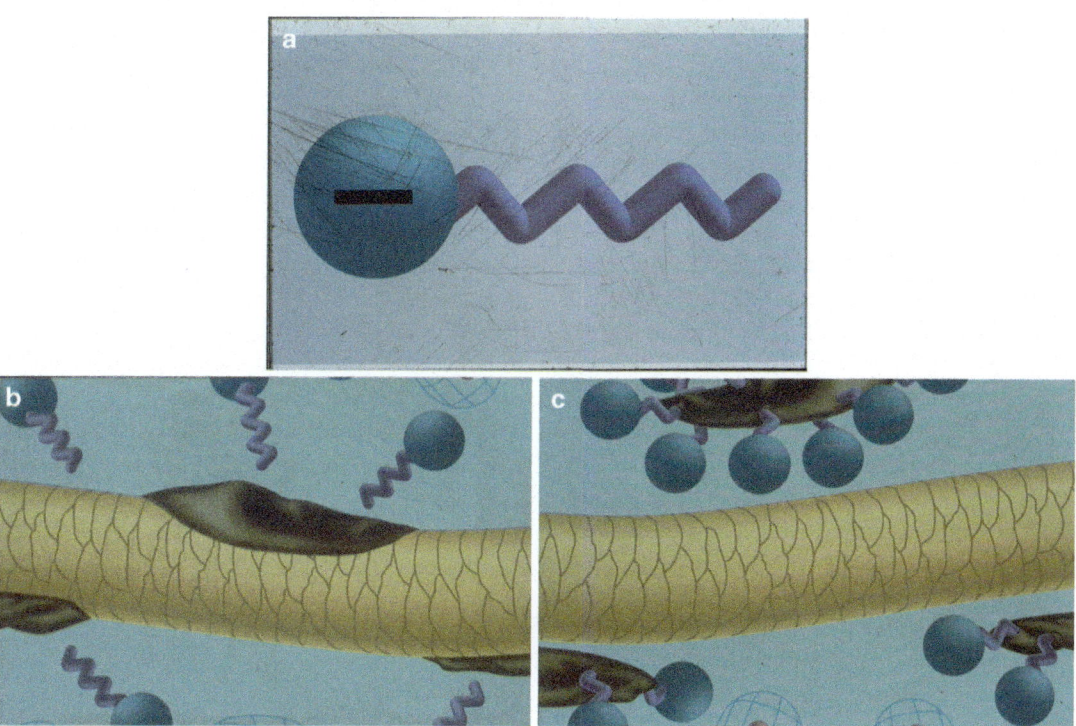

Fig. 7.6 (a) Surfactant molecule with hydrophilic head acts by (b) removing the dirt from the hair with a lipophilic (fat-loving) component and (c) transferring it to the rinse water with hydrophilic (water loving) component

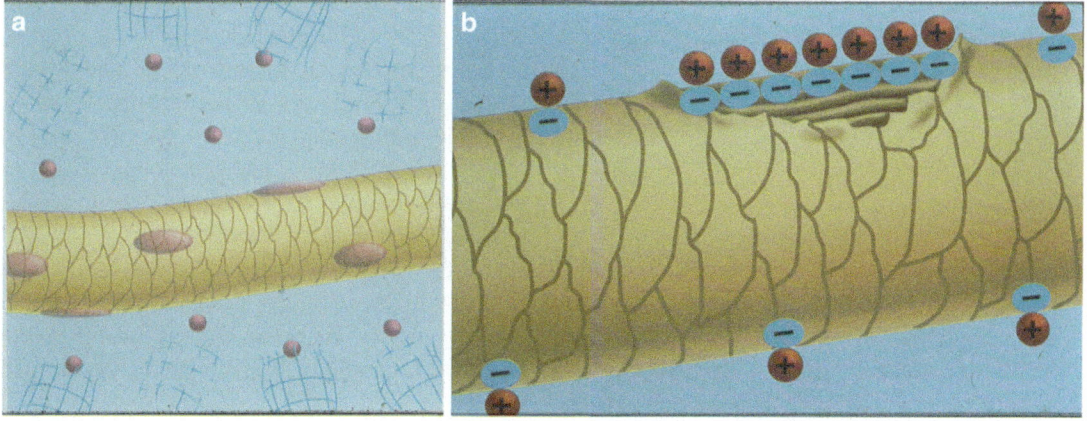

Fig. 7.7 (a, b) Deposition of silicones onto negatively charged surface of the damaged hair from a 2-in-1 product

Shampoos for Colour-Treated Hair

Over recent years, products have become more advanced in terms of efficiency of deposition of conditioning actives and also adjustment to different needs. Of particular interest has been shampoos and conditioners designed for women who colour and chemically treat their hair. Not only will these women potentially have more physical damage in terms of split ends, etc., but the efficiency of deposition of silicones such as dimethicones on coloured hair is significantly lower than on noncoloured hair.

This is driven by surface energy changes that occur during colouring and, specifically, the increase in surface hydrophilicity caused by loss of the surface bound f-layer lipid.

Polymers are also being used in shampoo formulations to enhance silicone deposition on previously coloured hair. As an example, a high-charge density polymer, poly(diallyldimethyl) ammonium chloride, on dilution forms a hydrophobic layer on hair, enhancing silicone deposition both from the shampoo itself and from the subsequent conditioner.

> **Science Box**
>
> Polymers
> A polymer is a large molecule (macromolecule) composed of many repeated subunits, known as monomers. Because of their broad range of properties, both synthetic and natural polymers are important in our daily lives. Polymers range from familiar synthetic plastics to natural biopolymers such as DNA and proteins. Polymers have a large molecular mass relative to their small molecular size, and they have unique physical properties including toughness and viscoelasticity. They are used in hair-care products for conditioning and styling purposes.

Conditioners

The concept of conditioning hair is not new. Essential oils (tea tree, jojoba) were used historically and continue to this day. The Victorians were keen on Macassar oil, and invented the anti-Macassar cover for chair backs to prevent greasy residues. Brilliantine is largely regarded as the first of modern conditioners, but was largely employed for softening moustaches.

The practice of regular conditioning after shampooing is relatively recent, and sadly, still not part of a global culture. In the light of worldwide colouring and bleaching, in addition to daily weathering, conditioning hair is critical to its sustained 'health' as it inevitably 'weathers' in an accelerated manner.

Early 'conditioners' were equivalent to greasy pomades and offered protection against the harsher effects of relaxers, permanents, straighteners, and colourants. Modern intensive conditioners can be formulated in a range from 'light' to 'heavy' and have much greater aesthetic properties. If used regularly, they can obviate the effects of chemical and physical processes.

Conditioner Mode of Action

A conditioning product deposits actives onto the surface of the hair shaft. It typically does this by creating a lamellar gel network structure composed of fatty alcohol and cationic surfactants with silicone suspended in the hydrophobic part of the gel network (Fig. 7.8a, b).

During the product application, the gel network spreads on hair, giving a very smooth feel, reducing knots and tangles. As the product then dries, the silicone spread evenly over the hair surface forming a thin layer and increasing surface hydrophobicity. This hydrophobic layer will change hair feel, especially when hair is dry, giving it a smooth, soft feel, and it will reduce hair friction and combing forces. Importantly, this will also reduce knot and tangle formation and reduce combing breakage.

Early silicone products were limited by the ability of formulators to include this type of technology into aqueous solutions. However, in the last 20 years, there has been an explosion in silicone technology such that one recent innovation has been the introduction of functionalised silicones such as terminal amino silicones (TAS), which add amine groups to the end of the silicone chains. By more closely matching the interfacial tension of the silicone to the surface energy of hair, the TAS silicone materials will deposit significantly better onto coloured and damaged hair than uncharged silicones, like dimethicone. These materials also have an additional benefit of improved ability to deposit on severely damaged hair tips than previous dimethicone silicones.

Different Conditioning Variants

The level of conditioning benefit can be increased by varying the levels and types of silicones and

Hair-Care Products for Different Hair Needs

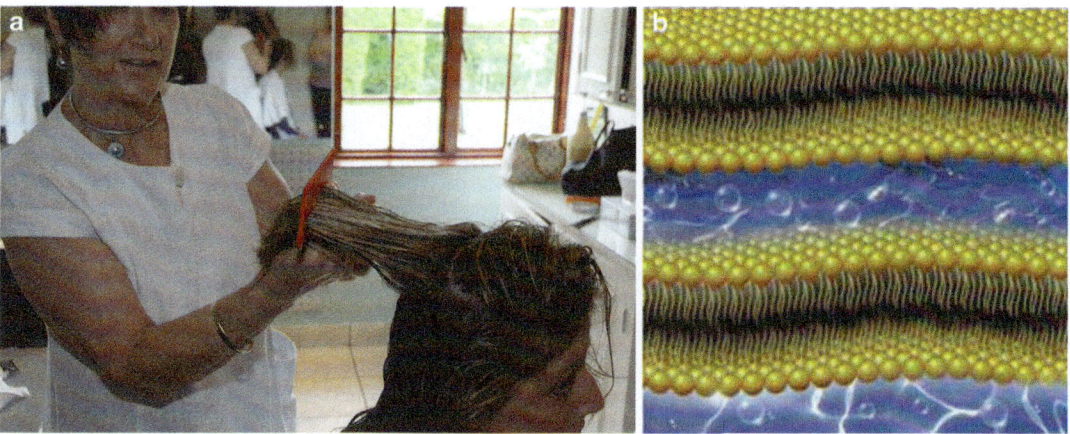

Fig. 7.8 (**a**) Combing conditioner through hair; (**b**) deposition of conditioning actives by creation of a lamellar gel network

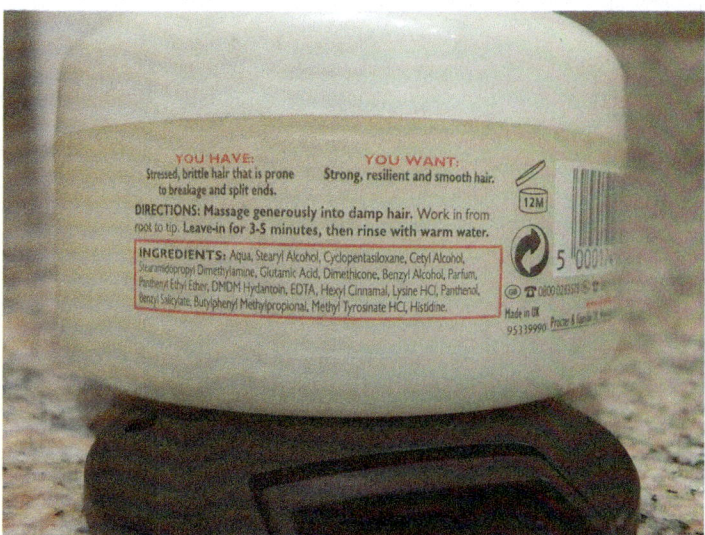

Fig. 7.9 Intensive conditioner. High levels of fatty alcohols (see ingredient listing) designed for significantly damaged hair

cationic surfactants used (in general, longer chain surfactants deliver higher conditioning).

Intensive conditioners are heavy and creamy in consistency since they contain high proportions of fatty alcohols and are well suited to hair that is significantly damaged or coarse. Such conditioners can be left in the hair for a long time and can temporarily hold split ends together (Fig. 7.9).

Leave-in conditioners tend to contain lighter weight conditioning materials, which add little weight to the hair. **Rinse-out conditioners** help control frizz and can help minimise the look of thinning hair (Fig. 7.10).

There are also 'hold' conditioners, which are combination products that provide the benefits of conditioning while also holding the hair in place like a mousse. This effect is achieved using cationic polymers.

Conditioning Products in Ethnic Usage

In Africa, many women who retain their natural phenotype employ light conditioning agents as their primary hair-care product. As the essential

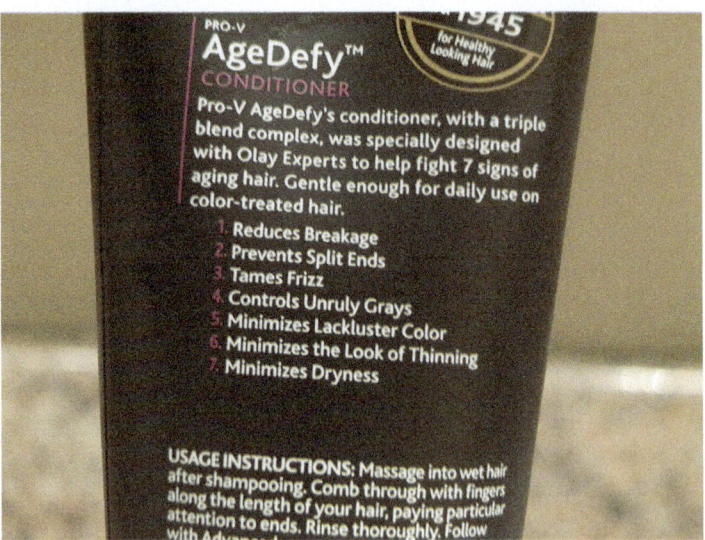

Fig. 7.10 Rinse-out conditioner, part of the regimen for thinning hair

need is for moisturisation rather than cleansing, this, by experience, is often their preferred method of hair care.

Oil Inclusion in Conditioning Products

Oils have a long history of use in hair care and are invariably culturally based. This history has driven the introduction of natural oils into modern hair-care products to deliver dry and wet feel benefits. In some cases, these ingredients supplement silicones. Examples of these oils include argan oil, Moroccan oil, and coconut oil.

Other ingredients in modern conditioners and hair-care preparations similarly work to smooth the outer layers of the cuticle. These may include protein extracts (collagen and the amino acids obtained from silk) and panthenol and similar compounds, which are related to vitamin B5. Some of these are known to penetrate into the cortex and to help to increase its moisture content. Keratin or hydrolysed keratin is another common ingredient added to products. Keratin proteins will typically not readily penetrate inside hair due to their large size. Hydrolysed keratins are more likely to penetrate, but neither active will replace lost proteins.

Key Ingredients of Conditioners

In Table 7.2, the key ingredients of conditioners are described, and the chemical names found on products are included.

Silicones

Silicones are an example of polymers and are now widely used as ingredients in hair conditioners, shampoos, and hair gel products. They are synthetic and chemically inert. Some silicones, notably the amine functionalised amodimethicones, are excellent conditioners, providing improved compatibility, feel, and softness and lessening frizz. The phenyltrimethicones are another silicone family and are used in reflection-enhancing and colour-correcting hair products, where they increase shine and glossiness.

Ethnic and Cultural Differences in Conditioning Preferences

The level of conditioning required to achieve optimum desired performance will depend on the hair phenotype and morphology (curl, diameter, etc.), hair style, and the level of hair damage. In general, women with European phenotype hair will tend to prefer lower-level conditioning

Hair-Care Products for Different Hair Needs

Table 7.2 Key ingredients of conditioners

Material class	Name to look for on products	Function
Silicone	Dimethicone, amodimethicone	Makes hair easier to comb, softer, and smoother
	Bis-aminopropyl dimethicone	Increases shine by increasing fibre to fibre alignment
Cationic surfactant	Stearamidopropyl dimethylamine, behentrimonium methosulfate, behentrimonium chloride, dicetyldimonium chloride	Positively charged molecules preferentially attracted to areas of damage. Makes hair easier to comb, softer, and smoother and less static
Fatty alcohol	Cetyl alcohol, stearyl alcohol	Gives hair a smooth feel when dry and improves wet combing
	Cetearyl alcohol (mix of cetyl and stearyl alcohol)	They give products a thick, creamy appearance
Oil/emollient	Hydrogenated coconut oil, mineral oil, argan oil, Moroccan oil	Moisturises hair to improve softness
Additional ingredients	Panthenol, vitamin E	Targeted benefits, e.g. moisturisation, antioxidant

products more suitable for their fine hair (Fig. 7.11). In contrast, women with hair of African descent tend to prefer high-level conditioning products that give high protection against knots and tangles (Fig. 7.12a, b). Indian and East Asian women also tend to prefer high conditioning benefits to drive a high shine and smooth look (Fig. 7.13a–c).

Special Hair Needs

Dry, woolly hair generally requires heavier deposits of conditioners than other hair types. The use of leave-in and 'intensive' conditioners is growing. The use of moisture-retaining ingredients (humectants) such as panthenol can be augmented by cationic ingredients (e.g. polyquaternium derivatives), which leave hair more manageable.

How to Select the Correct Hair-Care Regimen

One of THE major concerns women have regarding hair-care products is choosing the correct one for their hair type and style. Too low a conditioning level will not deliver the feel, shine, and frizz benefits they desire, but too high a conditioning level may create the possibility of weighed-down

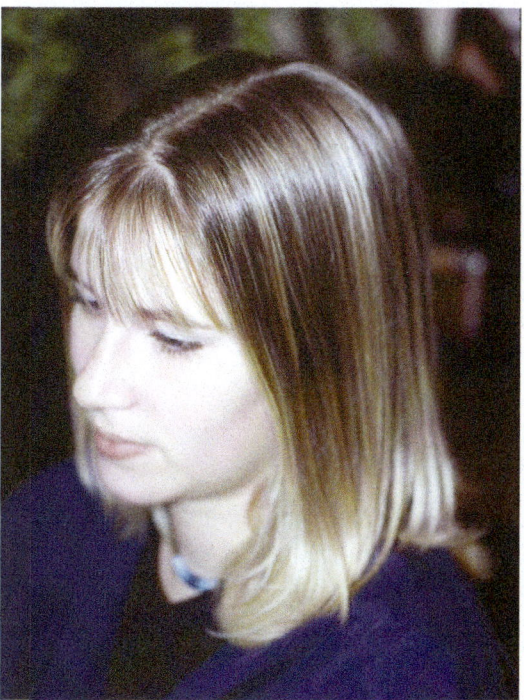

Fig. 7.11 In general, women with European phenotype hair will tend to prefer lower conditioning products more suitable for their fine hair

hair and a greasy, sticky feel and look. These negatives can be an issue when a high conditioning product is used on fine and/or straight hair.

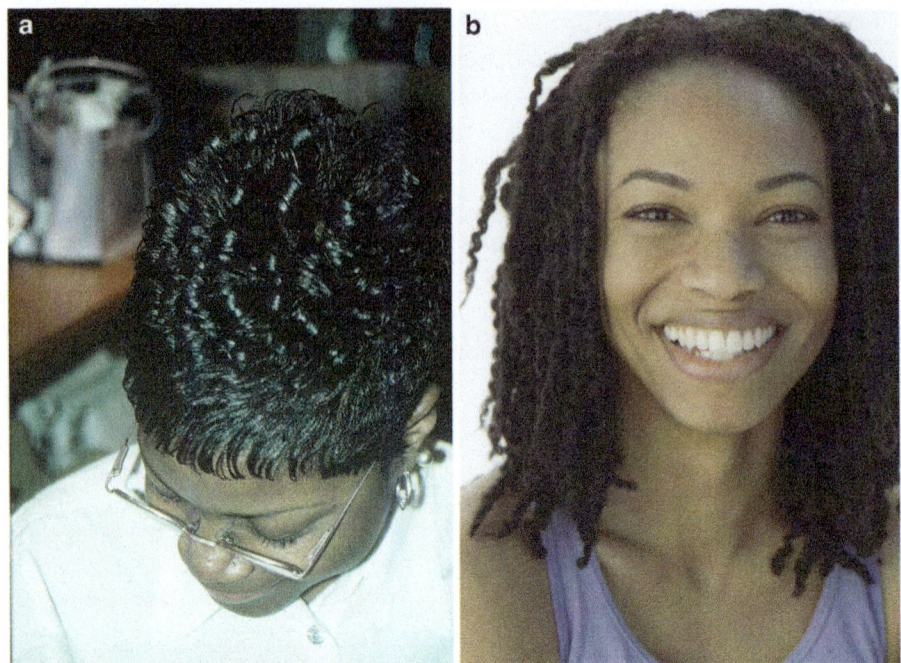

Fig. 7.12 (**a**, **b**) Women of African heritage tend to prefer high-level conditioning products that gives high protection against knots and tangles

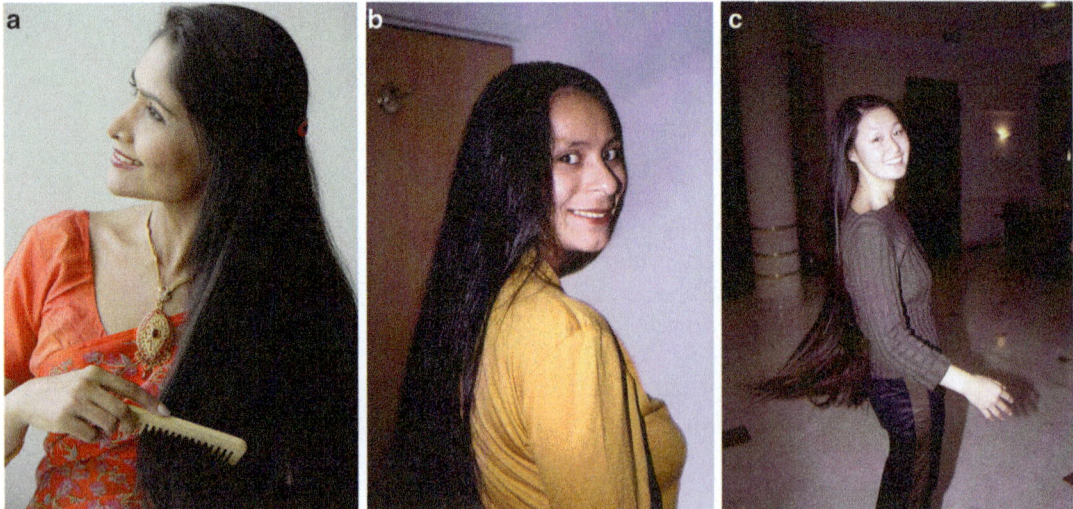

Fig. 7.13 (**a–c**) Indian and East Asian women also tend to prefer high conditioning benefits to drive a high shine and smooth look

To help women avoid these issues, product version names are being chosen to indicate a desired benefit, and the level of conditioning is commensurate with this and the assumed state of the hair.

Products may be labelled as a collection (regimen) under the following main benefit categories and from lowest to highest moisture capability:

- 'Volume'
- 'Clean'
- 'Defined curls'
- 'Smooth'
- 'Moisture'
- 'Strength/anti-breakage'
- 'Colour'
- 'Damage repair'

Within these broad categories will be a range of shampoos (including clarifying), conditioners of varying intensity, and styling products including mousses, gels, heat defence, hairsprays, and serums.

Volume

Women choosing this category tend to have finer, thinner hair texture or shorter length, desire more cleaning, and wash their hair more frequently (Fig. 7.14a, b). They tend to use a blow dryer, curling iron, and styling products to create and keep their desired look. Women state that they want to achieve healthy volume, but find their flat, lifeless hair is also prone to over-styling and over-conditioning.

'Volume' products tend to have low conditioning levels and contain polymers which add lift at the root. They are suitable for women with fine hair/low volume/undamaged hair.

Technical Solution

The technical solution for women requiring volume is to increase cleaning and lather cushion for detangling without depositing undue levels of conditioning agents on the hair. Consequently, products incorporate:

1. Higher surfactant levels to increase cleaning
2. Cationic polymer to improve lather cushion and detangling, but rinses clean to prevent deposition onto the hair
3. Low or no silicone to minimise deposition on the hair shaft in order not to weigh down the hair mass and to allow hair's own natural conditioning to provide volume

'Moisture' or 'Smooth'

Women seeking this benefit tend to have hair texture ranging from fine to coarse and would probably include hair which is dry with slight damage from heat and colouring. Such hair is susceptible to changes in humidity. Women desire an improvement in hair feel through balancing conditioning with cleaning. Shine is a requirement.

Products for these benefits are likely to have higher conditioning levels and are suitable for

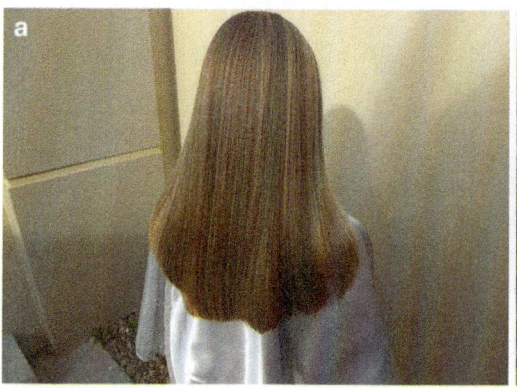
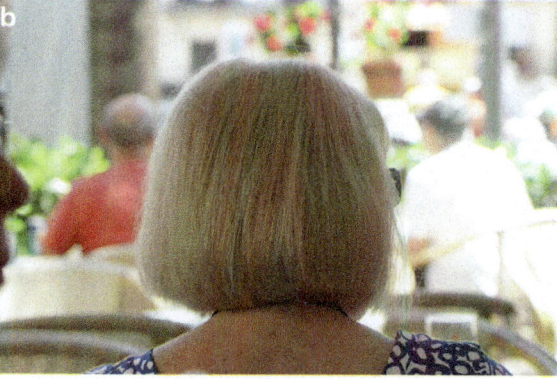

Fig. 7.14 Women with (**a**) finer, thinner hair texture and (**b**) with shorter length tend to wash their hair more frequently

Fig. 7.15 Products that moisturise and smooth hair are likely to have higher conditioning levels and are suitable for women with a degree of damage and a tendency to develop frizz and flyaway

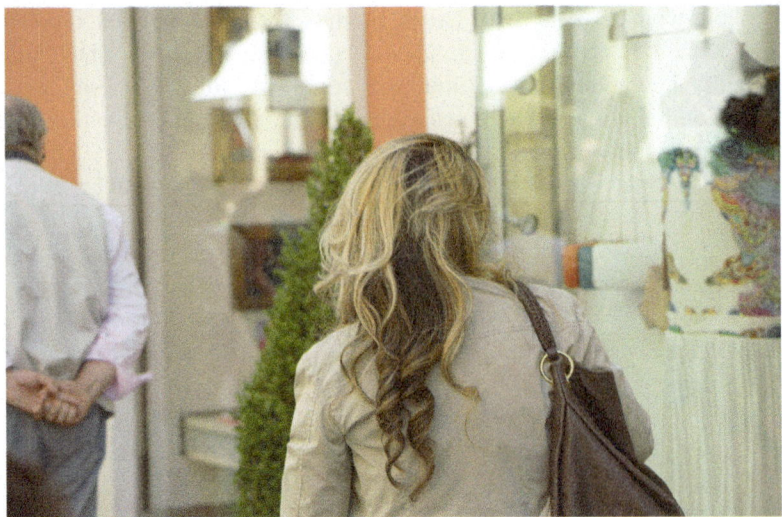

Fig. 7.16 Women with moderately unruly hair prone to dryness or frizz would normally find a variant in this category of products that provide moisture and smooth hair

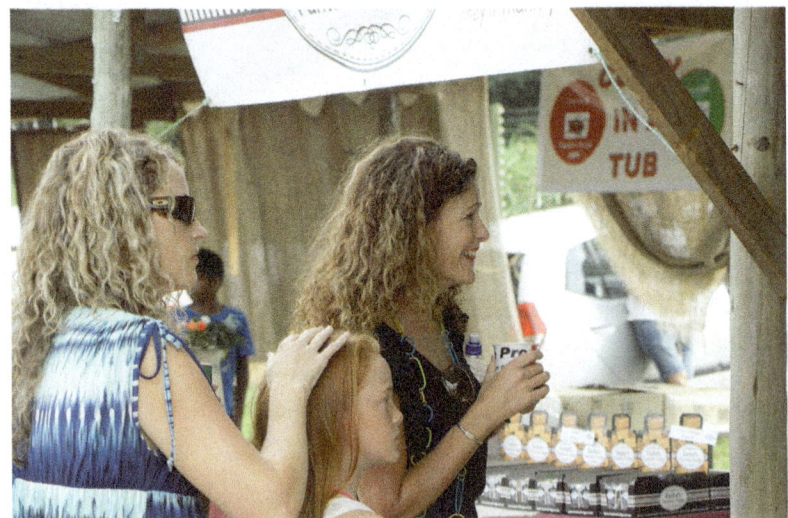

women with a degree of damage and a tendency to develop frizz and flyaway (Fig. 7.15). Women with unruly hair prone to dryness or frizz would normally find a variant in this category (Fig. 7.16).

Technical Solution

1. Higher molecular weight cationic polymer to provide more hair lubricity, detangling, and silicone deposition
2. Silicone which provides increased wet detangling and excellent dry conditioning with less weight on the hair
3. Oils are often added to minimise frizz and flyaway

'Damage Repair'

Women seeking this category of product tend to have hair with high levels of damage from overprocessing and over-styling (Fig. 7.17). They seek high conditioning levels from products, but also need sufficient cleaning, as they are likely to be using multiple steps. A technical challenge for this level of damaged hair is the strong negative charge it carries, so the deposition efficacy of silicone is low.

Practical Aspects of Hair Care

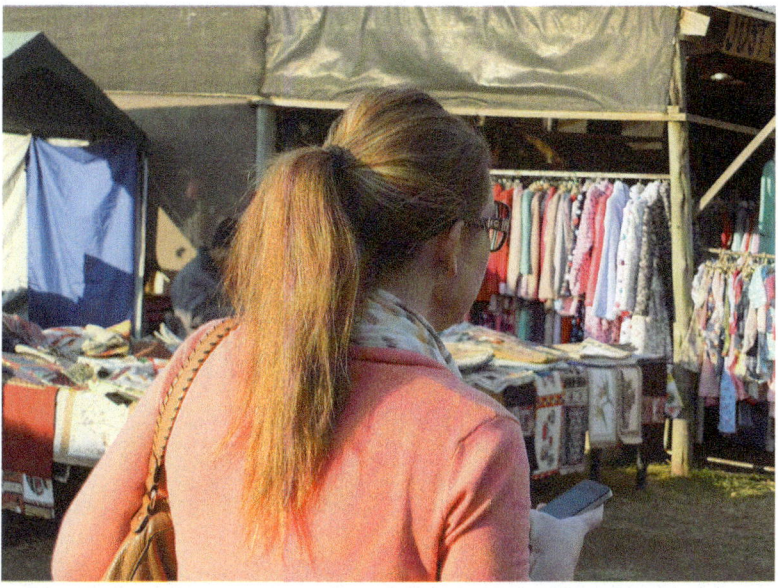

Fig. 7.17 Women who seek products offering 'damage repair' tend to have hair with high levels of damage from overprocessing and over-styling

These products will have the highest conditioning levels and are almost mandatory for women with repeated bleaching where the hair is fragile, porous, and prone to tangling and breakage. This category would include intense conditioners including 'masques', heat-defence serums, and potentially specialised products to manage severely damaged tips.

The different conditioning materials shown in Table 7.2 are generally specific to the product used to deliver the benefit.

Technical Solution

1. Higher level of cationic polymers to protect hair during washing and wet combing
2. Silicones to give high levels of dry conditioning and a moisturised, smooth feel

Other Product Categories

Other hair-care product categories will have carefully balanced cleansing and conditioning products aimed at addressing the prime concern of the woman, including:

- **Strength**: These products are designed for woman with a significant breakage problem.
- **Curls**: These products contain polymers which help define natural curls (Fig. 7.18).

Practical Aspects of Hair Care

In this section, some of the practical aspects of hair care with relevance to preserving hair health are described and illustrated, with examples from the home situation and in the salon.

Cleansing (Shampooing)

Washing Frequency

Many women ask their family, friends, stylist, and even doctor—'how often should I/can I wash my hair?' There is no scientific restriction on this frequency, and it is mostly dictated by habit, hair style, and time and in some cultures by water availability and economic circumstance. The frequency with which individuals shampoo varies from more than once daily to once every 2 weeks to never (Fig. 7.19a, b).

Signs of Need for Washing

Women judge whether their hair needs washing by both look and feel. If hair appears lank, has lack of volume, and is difficult to style, these are key indicators. Textural differences due to build-up of sebum and products, similarly so. Environment may play a part, with hot, humid conditions driving shampooing more than cold and/or dry. Social influences are also major influ-

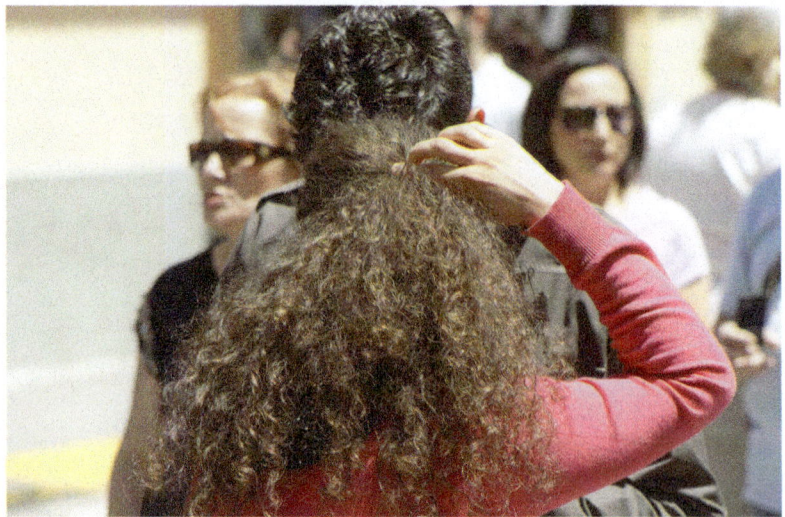

Fig. 7.18 Products containing polymers help define even the most challenging of natural curls

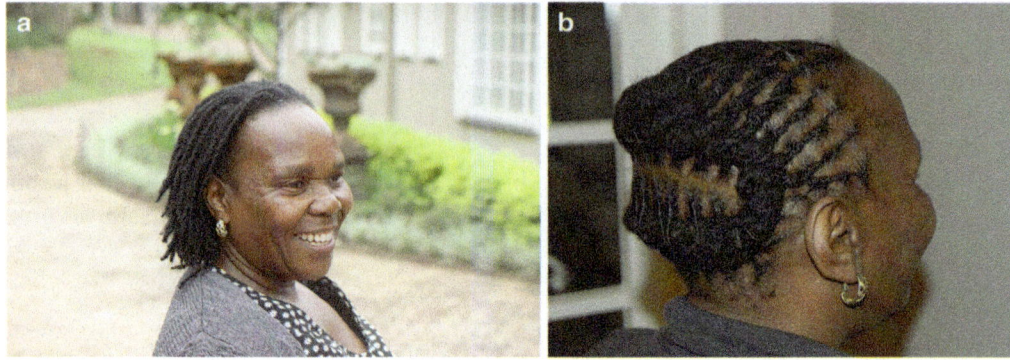

Fig. 7.19 (**a**, **b**) This lady in South Africa has her hair washed once every 2 weeks in a salon and invariably has dreadlocks attached or complex braiding afterwards

encers—no bride would approach the altar without serious attention to her hair.

Some women never wash their own hair. There is a strong tradition of the weekly 'wash and set' among senior citizens which consists of the use of curlers and or blow drying.

Step by Step: Shampooing

In this section, we offer some practical tips on how to achieve maximum benefit from a shampoo. First, select from the range that most suits the hair phenotype and end benefit needs. In the salon, the backwash and an operative make life easier for the client, but the principles of shampooing are identical: to remove sebum, detritus, and styling products. In the sequence seen in Fig. 7.20a, b, the first lady has a substantial hair mass of fine, naturally blonde hair, worn to the nape of the neck. She has never processed her hair and washes it at least every other day, guided by look, feel, and social necessity. She only needs very light conditioning, but spends considerable time styling wherein she uses a number of products and implements to obtain her desired look.

The other lady has longer hair which has been heavily processed and is considerably damaged. She still has highlights and, in order to rectify the damage, has been using conditioning products at home before visiting a top stylist for a cut and style.

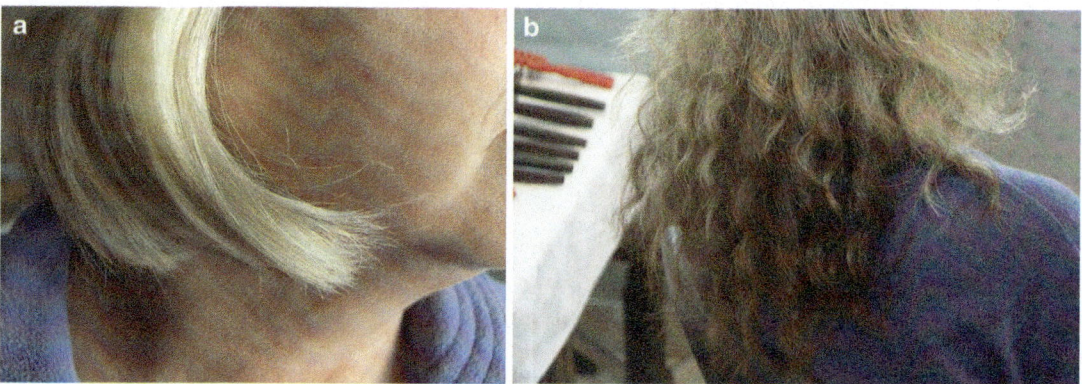

Fig. 7.20 Signs that hair needs washing: (**a**) clumping of the tips and (**b**) the hair mass as a whole needs washing in order to cut and style

Fig. 7.21 Measure the shampoo into the hand

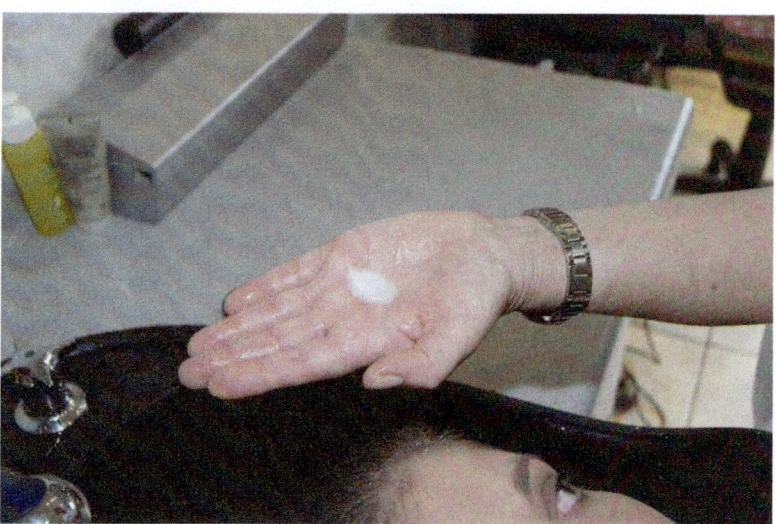

General Tips

- Women with long or curly hair should gently comb or brush the hair before wetting—starting from the tips and working up with a wide-toothed comb or brush.
- Gently wet the hair with warm water, working upwards with the hands if hair is long or curly.
- Measure the shampoo into one palm and spread the product evenly across both palms (Figs. 7.21 and 7.22).
- Gently work the shampoo into the hair starting at the roots and working down the hair to the tips (Fig. 7.23a, b).
- Do NOT pile hair on the head; this increases tangling.
- Rinse thoroughly with warm water, which has been shown to give more shine than cold (Fig. 7.24a, b).
- Repeat if no foam remains after shampoo has been thoroughly distributed.

Step by Step: Conditioning

Conditioning is done far less frequently than shampooing in every region. Sadly, many women do not realise how important it is for hair health.

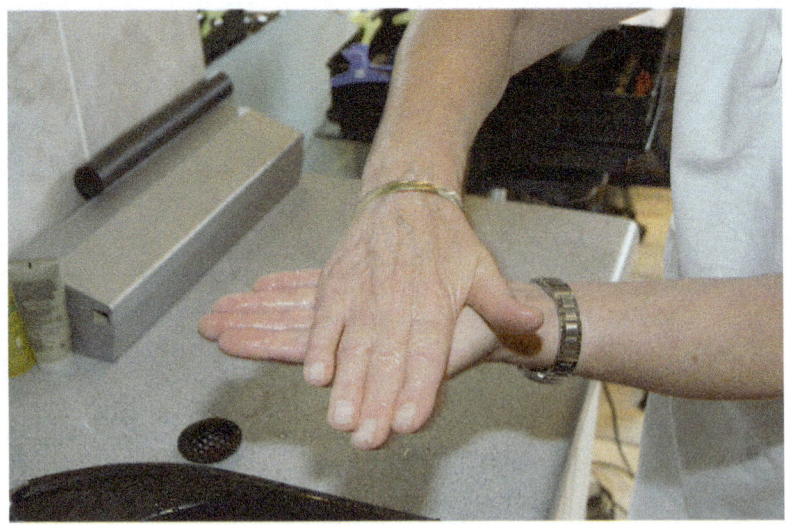

Fig. 7.22 Spread the shampoo evenly across both hands

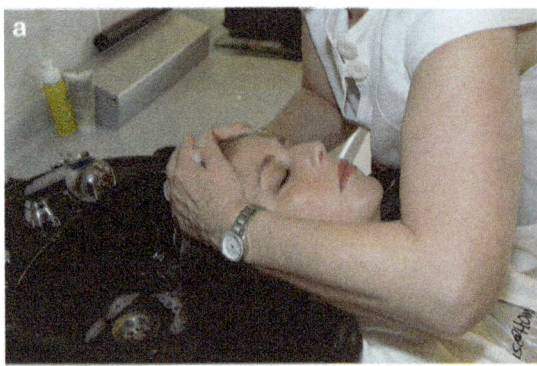
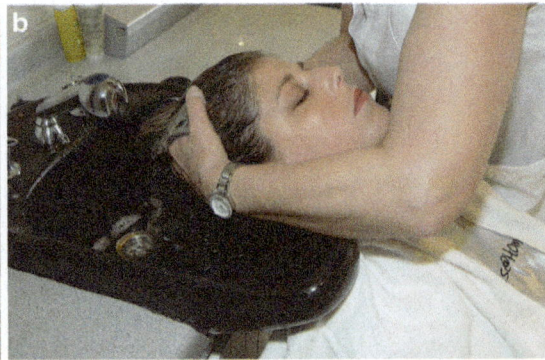

Fig. 7.23 Apply shampoo (**a**) gently working from the scalp down, spreading with the fingers across the scalp and (**b**) down the hair. Repeat process if hair has much styling product or is long or hair has not been washed for several days. A signal for a required repeat of shampoo application is low or no foam after shampoo is distributed

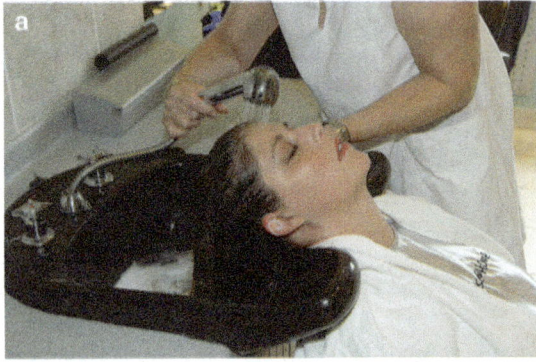
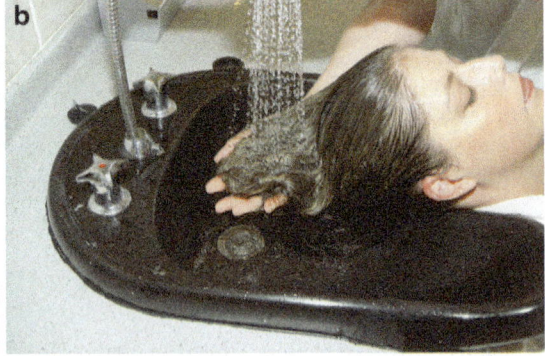

Fig. 7.24 (**a**) Rinse thoroughly with **warm** water, (**b**) working from scalp down. Do not cold rinse. Warm rinse produces a better shine result

Regular conditioning reduces tangling, static, and frizz and ultimately allows women to achieve volume control and voluminous styles.

The need to condition and the amount and type of conditioning required is governed by both feel and look. In addition, prevention is better than attempting to repair damage once it has occurred. There are some imperative situations where conditioning is mandatory. These include any recent chemical procedure such as bleaching, colouring, perming, or relaxing. Swimming or excessive sun exposure is another key driver.

Intensive conditioners or 'masques' may be used at least weekly for hair which is very damaged. These are presented in the regimens such as 'damage repair' and are designed to be left in for a prolonged period. The tips of the hair will always tend to need immediate intensive conditioning. However, attention to the mid shaft and even higher is important to prevention or reduction of damage. Even 'virgin' hair and women wanting volume warrant conditioning to prevent damage, particularly if it is to be worn long.

General Tips

- Select the conditioner from the range appropriate to the hair phenotype.
- Disperse the conditioner across the hands (Fig. 7.25)
- Apply the product first to the tips of the hair (Fig. 7.26).
- Unlike shampooing, start at the tips and work up the hair using the fingers. For severely damaged tips, leave conditioner on for 10 min (Fig. 7.27).
- Gently separate hair using fingers or a wide-tooth comb to ensure conditioner is fully distributed (Fig. 7.28).
- Rinse the hair well with warm water (Fig. 7.29).

Summary

Conditioning materials are formulated as emulsions and are traditionally applied after shampooing to increase hair 'quality' before grooming. They reduce negative charge, prevent flyaway, and increase manageability, thus reducing tangling. Other ingredients are classed as humectants—essentially they have the ability to increase moisture content and minimise moisture movement in and out of the hair.

Modern, high-quality conditioners increase the manageability, shine, and moisture content of each hair shaft and are designed to provide one or more of the following functions:

- Increase the ease of wet and dry combing
- Smooth, seal, and realign damaged areas of the hair shaft

Fig. 7.25 Disperse conditioner across the hands

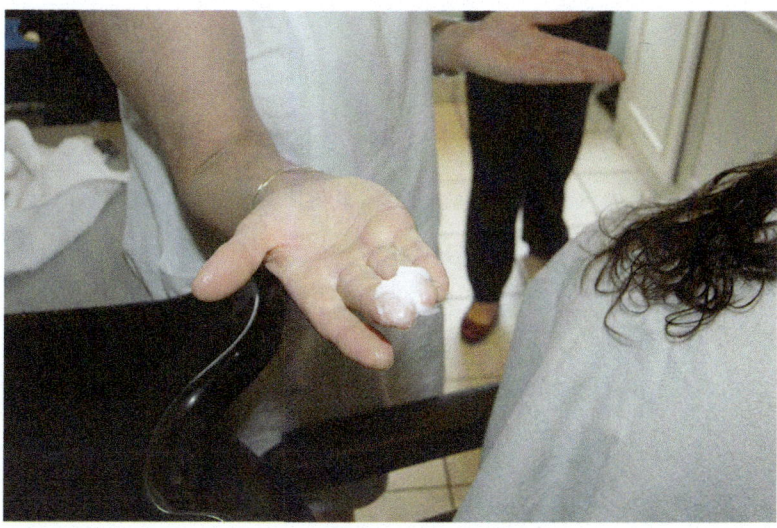

Fig. 7.26 Apply to the tips of hair first

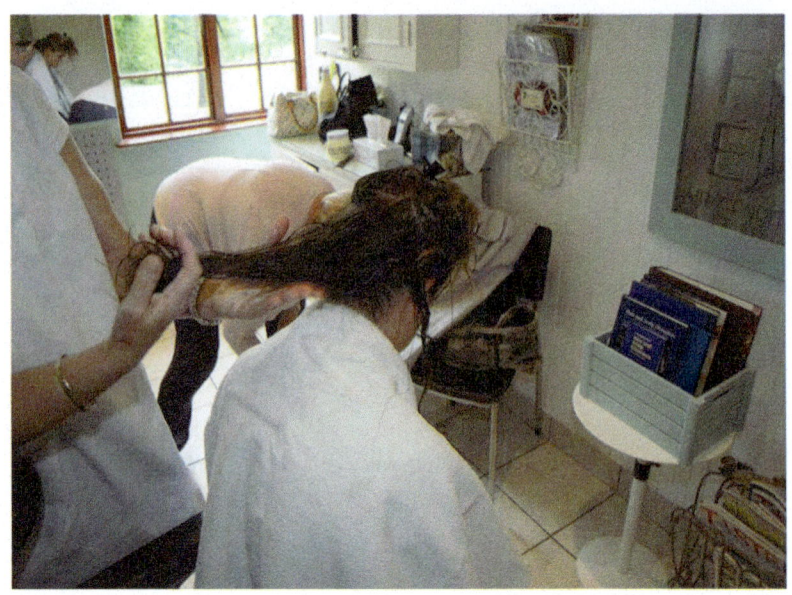

Fig. 7.27 Work up the hair, using the fingers

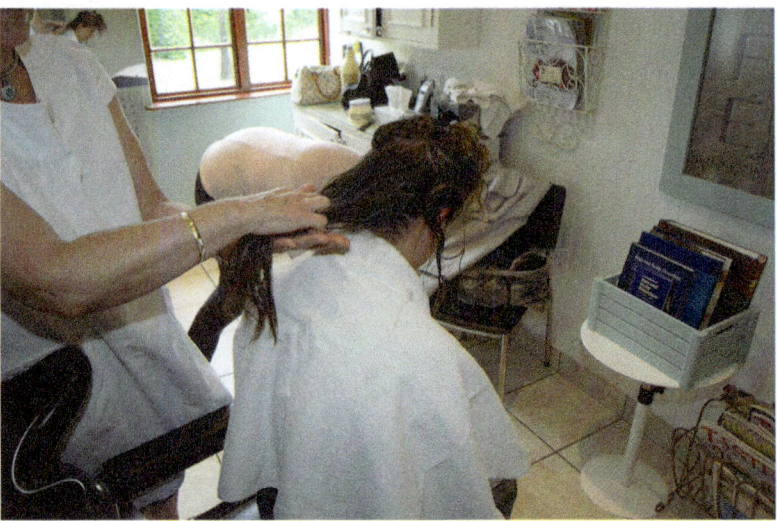

Fig. 7.28 Using a wide-tooth comb ensures that the conditioner is fully distributed

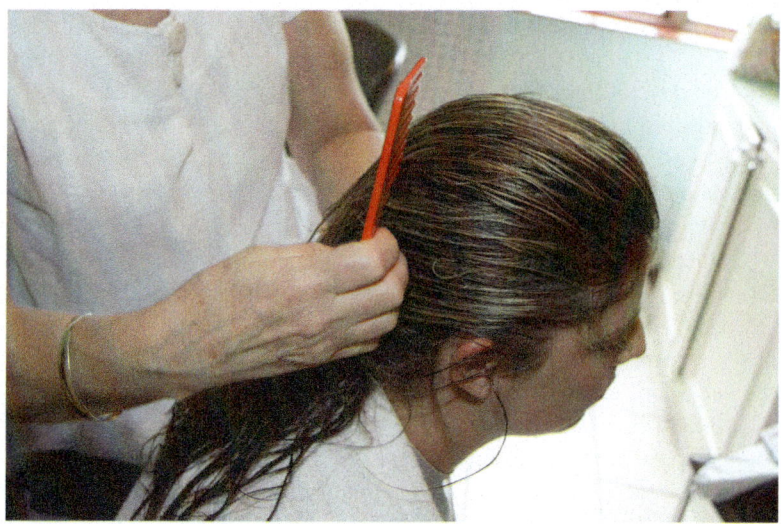

Fig. 7.29 Rinse well

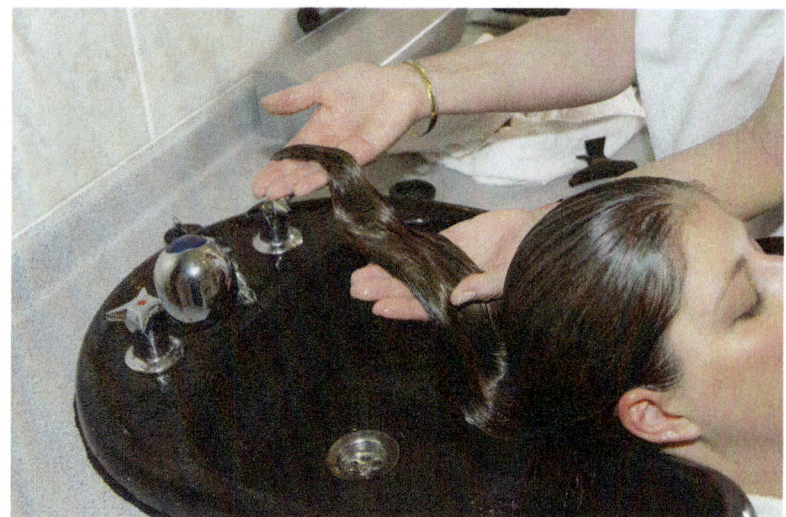

- Minimise porosity
- Impart sheen and a silken feel to hair
- Provide some protection against thermal and mechanical damage
- Moisturise
- Add volume and body
- Eliminate static electricity

Styling and Hair Health

For most women around the world, a 'good' cut utilising the intrinsic nature of the hair and its patterns is the first essential step for good style. Prior to this is the necessity for cleansing and regular conditioning, particularly if the hair is subjected to repeated insults as described in Chap. 3.

Each day, millions of women strive to achieve their desired style for work and recreation. In order to do this, they may employ nothing other than natural drying or, alternatively, a wide range of implements and products.

The application of physical forces on the hair (combing, brushing, teasing, backcombing) and the use of heat (natural or forced drying, direct heat) have potentially serious consequences for the hair shaft, especially since these actions will most likely be repeated thousands of times. The judicious use of moisturising detanglers and heat protection sprays can improve the quality and integrity of the hair shafts and help in the preservation of hair health.

In this section, the technologies behind these products are described, and a practical guide to their use is offered.

Styling Problems

Of all the various issues with hair styling, time and the intrinsic nature of each woman's hair are the most problematic. Hair phenotype dictates very largely what is easily achieved. Whatever the issue, modern hair-care products applied correctly and regularly can contribute significantly to the improvement of these situations.

Certain hair phenotypes have inherent problems—Classical Northern European hair is very fine and tends to lankness and lack of body. Very curly dry hair suffers from physical grooming problems. Indian and Oriental women typically desire a smooth and sleek look, but many have a considerable hair mass and even significant wave, which requires excessive amounts of time to manage. Wavy or very curly Caucasian hair suffers from frizz and flyaway and needs products to control.

Volume Control

Control of 'volume' is the most common driver for 'styling'. Volume in the broadest sense implies either too little or too much (Fig. 7.30a–c). It may be the desire to increase volume for those with fine or thinning hair. Alternatively, it may be the control of wayward curls. It is the desire to control volume and keep it in a day-long style which is the ultimate end benefit for millions of women.

The key factors affecting volume are:

- Diameter
- Density
- Stiffness
- Friction
- Cohesion

For women with fine to medium hair who desire to **increase** or **control** volume, there are a number of strategies which, in combination with styling and heat protection products, can produce the desired end benefit.

Blow Drying

With the introduction of precision cutting techniques in the 1970s, blow drying became universally popular in the salon and at home. The blow dryer works by using a heated air flow (up to ~80 °C) to first rapidly remove water held between hair strands. It then evaporates water from inside each hair strand, at which point the hair can be shaped into the desired style, forming a 'wet set'. The wet set is improved by evaporating as much water as possible, and inadequate drying is one reason why style does not hold. How long the wet set will keep its style during the day depends to some extent on the temperature and humidity. At high relative humidity, moisture in the air will penetrate hair, breaking temporary hydrogen binds holding the style in place, and hair will revert back to its natural shape (Fig. 7.31a, b).

Flat/Curling Irons

Flat irons or curling irons are also used to achieve the desired volume. These implements can reach temperatures up to 220 °C and are effective at removing water and creating a very effective wet set. However, these implements can cause significant damage, especially if used at a high temperature

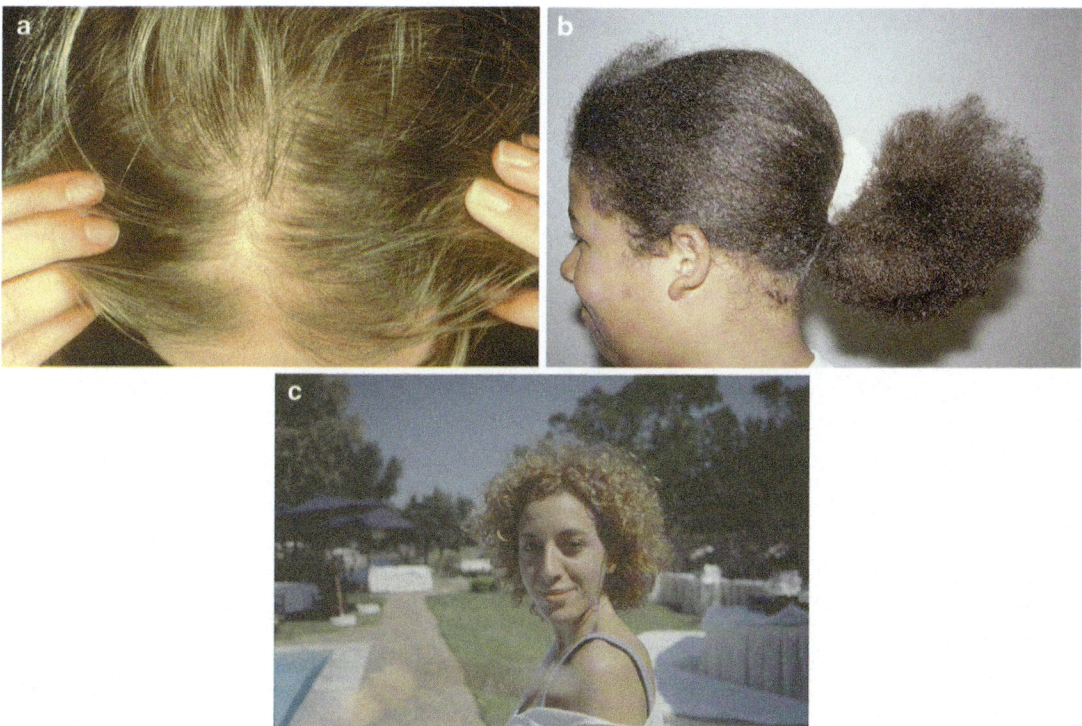

Fig. 7.30 Three volume problems: (**a**) not enough, (**b**) too much, and (**c**) managing curls

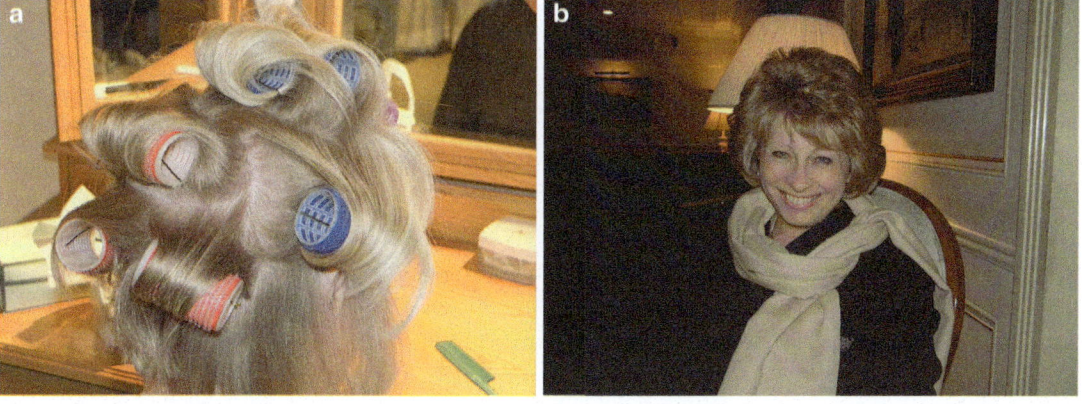

Fig. 7.31 Fine hair showing volume created by (**a**) blow drying and rollers, styling products, and hairspray. Time is also a requirement in order to create (**b**) a day-long style

setting or used for an excessive amount of time. Care should be taken to keep the heat setting below 190 °C and limit the number of passes (Fig. 7.32).

Heat protection products can help reduce damage by smoothing the hair surface, making it easier to pass the flat iron through hair and reduce localised heating.

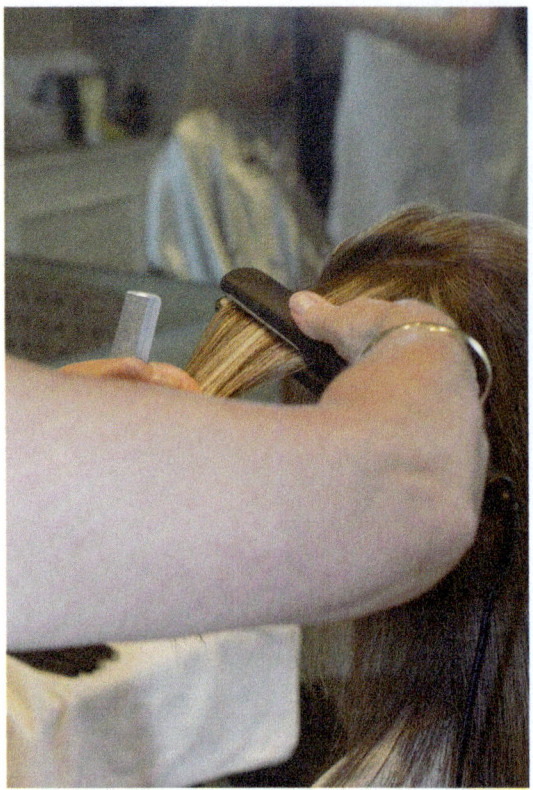

Fig. 7.32 The temperatures generated by some implements, such as hair dryers and hot combs, can exceed 200 °C and may cause significant hair damage

Temporarily Increasing Hair Fiction

There are three ways of temporarily increasing friction, which also helps to increase volume and fullness:

1. **Cleaning**—Hair's natural oils or sebum can build up over time, making hair more slippery, reducing friction, and making hair limp. Cleaning these oils off with a volume-building shampoo will restore hair's natural tendency to volume.
2. **Teasing**—Teasing, or combing hair backwards, from tip to root will roughen the cuticle, drastically increasing friction. This temporarily creates volume, but is potentially very damaging over time. Teasing causes the cuticle layers to roll and peel up (Fig. 7.33a, b).
3. **Styling products**—These products can create stiffness at the root to create volume. Spacer particles can also be added to provide volume by separating fibres.

Straightening

There are several ways to straighten hair, depending on the starting level of curl and how permanent the treatment is. As permanency increases, there are also trade-offs with hair health because these treatments involve reactive chemistry that can impact fibre integrity.

The least permanent way to straighten hair is blow drying and/or flat ironing, as discussed previously. This method uses heat to create a wet set, which will only last until the next wash. Using excessive heat (>190 °C) can be detrimental to hair health, as will be excessive use of such implements.

A recent popular straightening treatment is keratin treatments such as Brazilian keratin treatment. These products use formaldehyde to cross-link hair into a straight shape. The active is applied, and then cross-linking is activated by heat during the flat-ironing final step. The formaldehyde-containing products have become less common in the last few years as regulations have restricted its use globally due to safety concerns. Alternative products are emerging, including those containing glyoxylic acid and glyoxyloyl carbocysteine, which work via a similar cross-linking mechanism. There have been reports of these products causing hair breakage, which could either be due to the high flat iron temperatures used to create the original style or repeated treatments where multiple cross-links eventually make hair very brittle and easy to break. Cross-link products are more effective for women with wavy hair vs. very curly hair, and typically last 2–3 months, depending on wash frequency.

An alternative for women with curlier hair is Japanese straightening treatment. The products, which have been in the market from many years, employ thioglycolate technology to straighten hair prone to frizz. Care must be taken when applying the thioglycolate chemistry, as it can irreversibly damage hair by breaking down the disulphide bonds which give hair its strength if

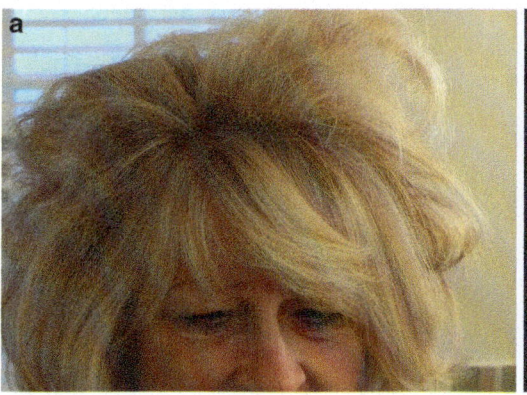 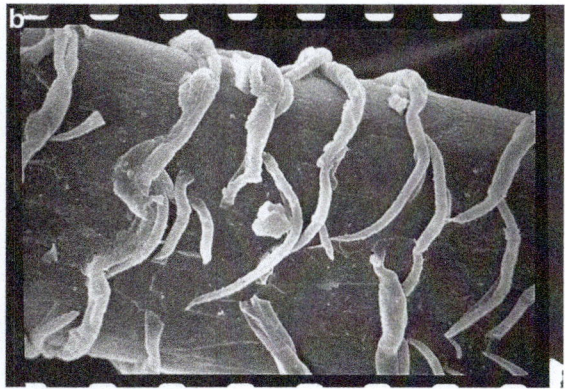

Fig. 7.33 (a) Teasing or combing hair backwards from tip to root will (b) roughen the cuticle, drastically increasing friction

left too long on the hair. Typically, this chemistry is best applied in the salon by experts who can accurately judge processing time and get the optimum result. These products will work well on women with wavy and curly hair and will last 3–6 months. However, they generally will not be able to fully straighten highly curly hair.

For women with highly curled hair, e.g. women of African descent, straightening is achieved with relaxer treatments (Fig. 7.34a–c). Most relaxers are high pH products in the form of heavy creams consisting of very high oil-in-water emulsions which are combed through the hair, where they slowly break down the structural bonds. The aggressiveness of the caustic is controlled by the incorporation of suitable emollient oils. The two most common types of relaxers are sodium hydroxide (lye) and guanidine hydroxide (no lye). Also on the market are potassium and lithium hydroxide relaxers as well as ammonium bisulphite relaxers. However, sodium hydroxide and guanidine hydroxide have proven to be the most effective. Guanidine hydroxide relaxers are considered less irritating to the scalp than lye-based relaxers; therefore, some women prefer them. No-lye products, although considered less harsh, can still burn the scalp, eyes, and ears.

Relaxers are the most damaging to hair structure of all the straightening products, but they are also the most permanent and effective. Relaxed hair thus requires considerable aftercare. Modern hair-care products have been developed for this market, and the conditioners include fatty alcohols and light mineral oils to maintain the critical moisture content.

Styling Products

A range of styling products to create long-lasting styles has emerged to complement the new generation of cleansing and conditioning products. These can enhance or alter most common aesthetic styling problems. Foremost among these is the control of 'volume', either too little or too much. Managing frizzy hair is important, too, and products for the so-called ethnic hair are emerging.

Styling products help keep long-lasting volume by creating reinforcing bonds between hair shafts at critical locations to the style. These bonds come in two types:

- **Seam welds**—Seam welds are bonds created that hold two hair shafts together in side-by-side alignment.
- **Spot welds**—Spot welds are found where hairs cross each other to create a support structure (Fig. 7.35). The styling polymer glues the shafts together at this critical structural point.

Hairspray

Hairspray (also hair lacquer or spritz) is sprayed onto dry hair to keep it stiff or in a certain style. The spray can be dispensed from a pump or

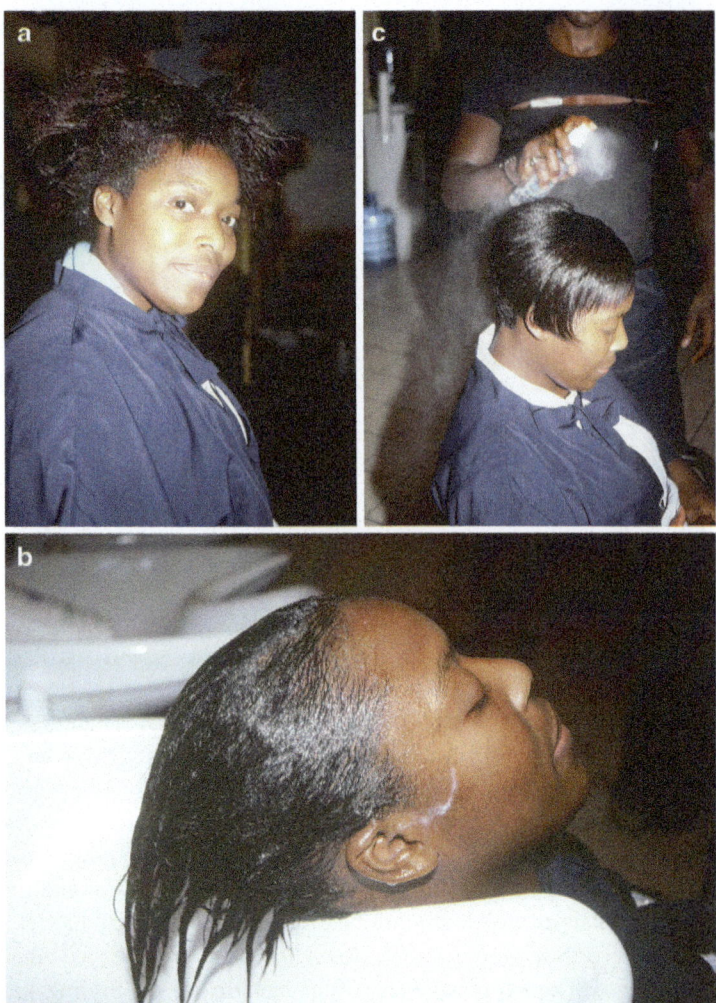

Fig. 7.34 (a) For women with highly curled hair, a relaxer works best for straightening. (b) Most relaxers are formulated in the form of heavy creams consisting of very high oil-in-water emulsions which are combed through the hair where they slowly break down the structural bonds. (c) Relaxed hair allows for easier grooming

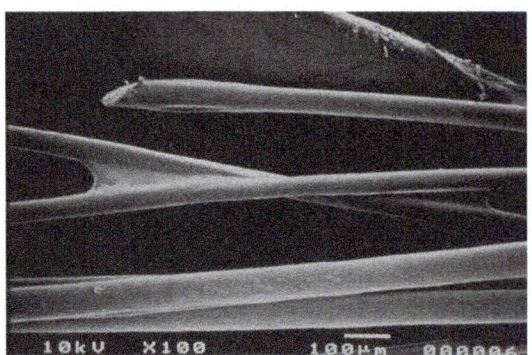

Fig. 7.35 Spot welds are found where hairs cross each other to create a support structure. The styling polymer glues the shafts together at this critical structural point

aerosol spray nozzle. Modern hairsprays were developed around the time of the aerosol can in the 1940s.

Hairspray is the most common styler and is a solution of polymer in a mixture of solvents and propellants that is sprayed on the hair in droplets. The droplets are formed when the liquid is forced through a pinhole in the nozzle of the can. In aerosol hairsprays, the force is supplied by propellant. In non-aerosols, the force is supplied via mechanical action of pumping the nozzle. Typically, non-aerosol's propellants provide more force than mechanical pumping, resulting in smaller droplet sizes. Smaller droplets dry faster, giving aerosol hairspray a 'drier' feeling than non-aerosol hairspray.

Ingredients are a blend of polymers that provide structural support to hair and include copolymers of polyvinylpyrrolidone (PVP) and polyvinyl acetate (PV). This copolymer mixture is usually modified to achieve the desired physical properties (adhesive strength, foaming, etc.). As the product dries, the polymer forms spot welds to hold the desired style in place.

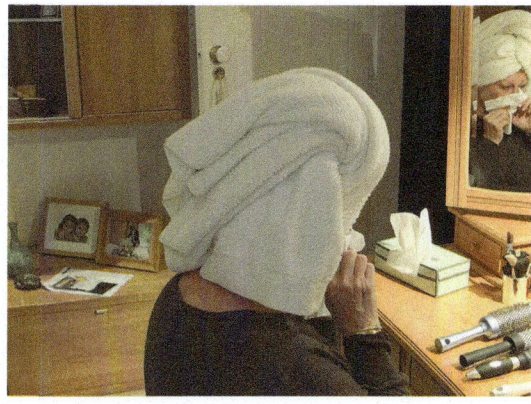

Fig. 7.36 Dry hair with loose towel

Mousse

Mousses are typically added to wet hair before styling. They use a propellant and a surfactant in addition to water-soluble styling polymers to create a smooth, creamy foam which is easy to spread through hair. The hair is then blow-dried, and the polymers form spot and seam welds to hold the style.

Hair Gels/Waxes/Pomades

These products are typically added to dry hair and are popular with men and women with short hairstyles. They can hold hair in different shapes and create, for example, a 'wet' or a 'textured' look. They contain polymers and high levels of waxes which hold the hair in place.

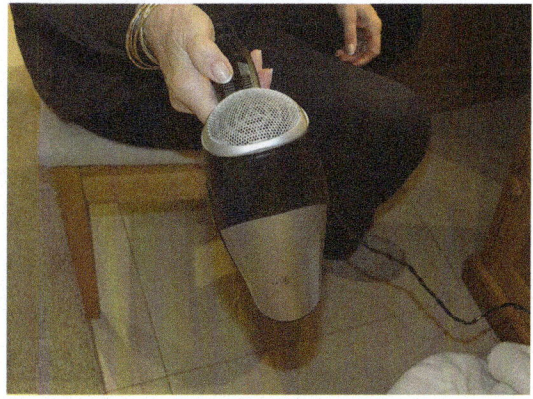

Fig. 7.37 Select medium temperature on the blow dryer

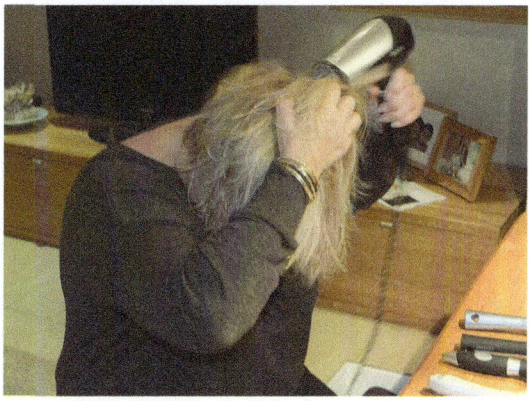

Tips for Healthy Styling

Once the hair has been cleansed and conditioned, it is now prepared for the creation of the desired style. This takes time. Hair is better able to hold a style if it is dried carefully and, preferably, slowly. Planning the process is important. In the same manner, as we have recommended conditioning from the tips to the roots, the same applies to drying and styling:

Fig. 7.38 Gently dry hair mass

- Gently dry hair with a loose towel (Fig. 7.36).
- Select a quality blow dryer and use a medium setting; dry the hair gently until it is barely damp (Figs. 7.37 and 7.38).
- Use a styling product of your choice (mousse, styling lotion, or spray) for the desired end benefit, and gently work into the hair with the fingertips (Fig. 7.39a–c).
- Apply a heat-defence product with the fingers (Fig. 7.40).
- Use a quality brush (circular or straight, depending on desired style) and finish drying

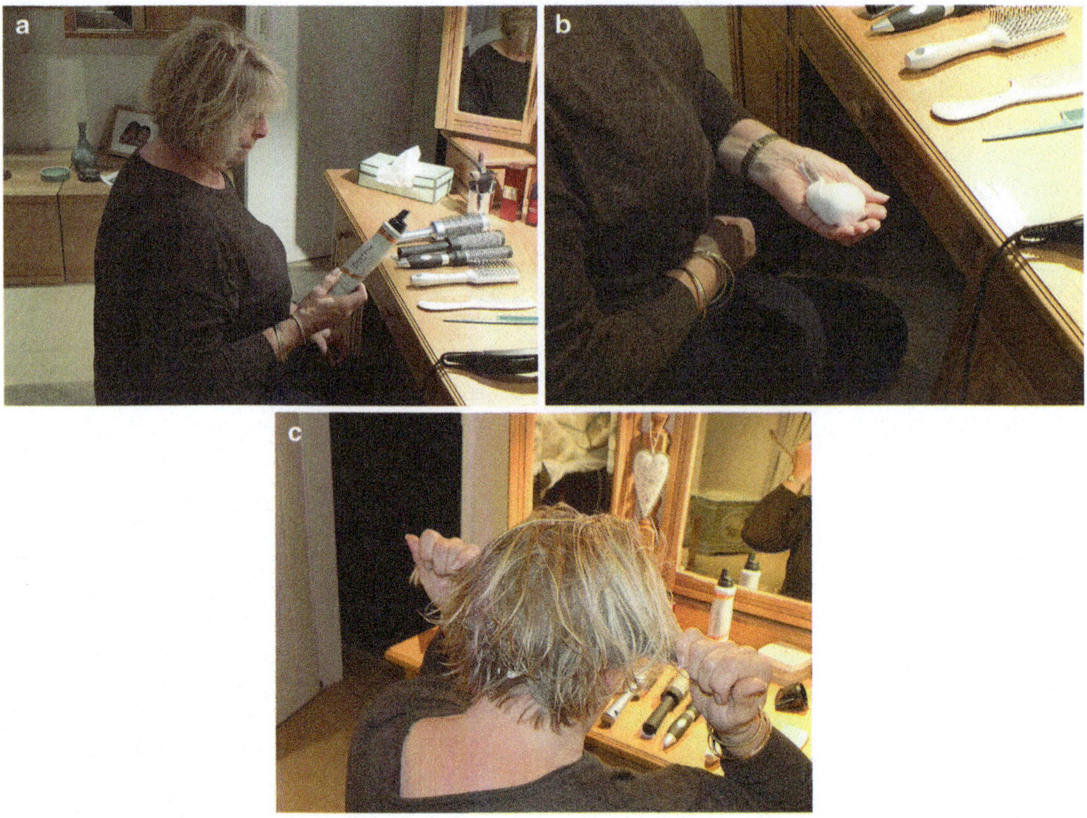

Fig. 7.39 (**a**) Select desired styling product for end benefit; (**b**) use proper amount; and (**c**) work into hair with hands

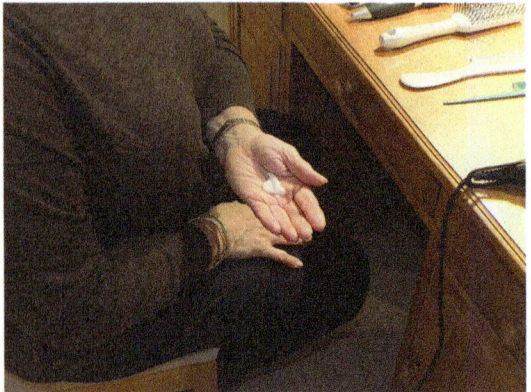

Fig. 7.40 Select heat-defence product

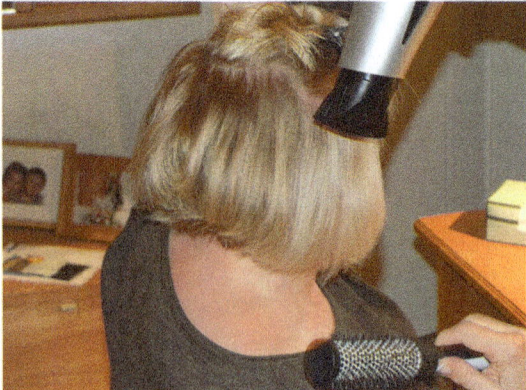

Fig. 7.41 Dry hair gently on medium setting, using circular brush to style

Summary

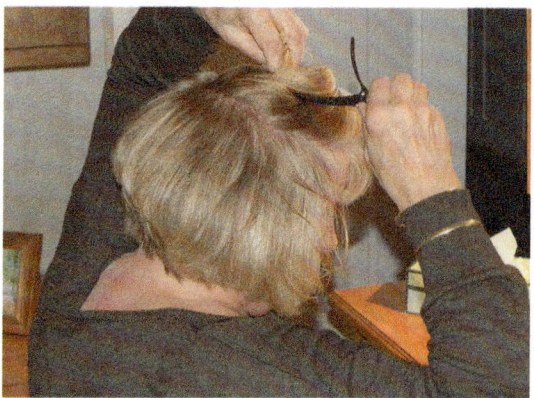

Fig. 7.42 Use clips to aid drying

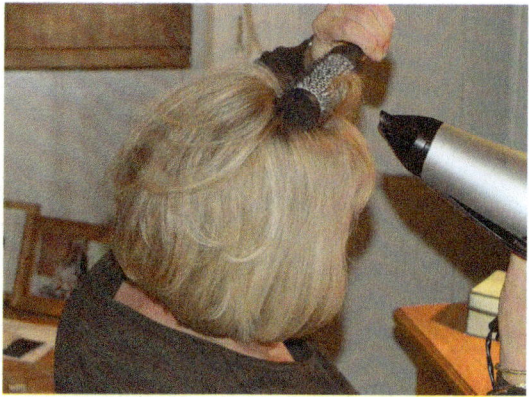

Fig. 7.43 Make sure each section is dry before moving on to the next

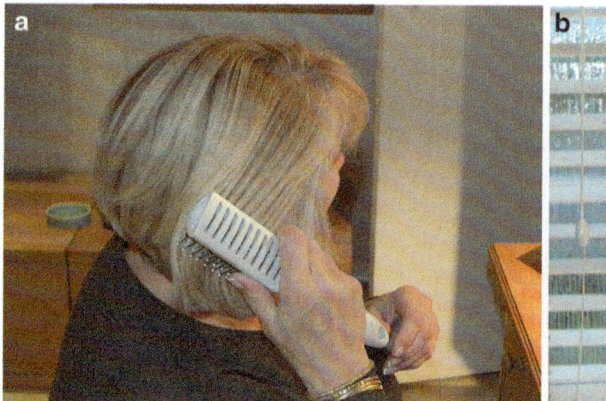
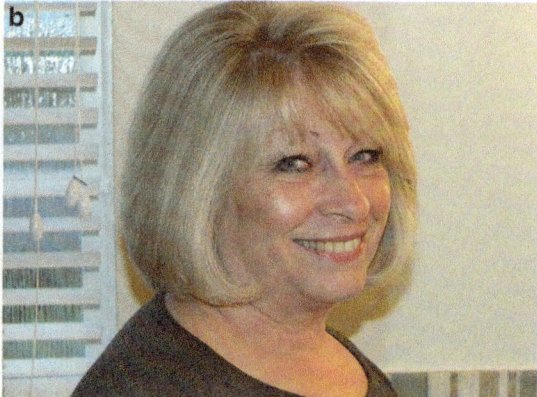

Fig. 7.44 (**a**) Smooth hair with wide brush and use (optional) hairspray for (**b**) day-long control

the hair, keeping the dryer a distance from the hair (Fig. 7.41).
- Segment the hair with clips to enable it to be dried in the so-called triangular manner (Fig. 7.42).
- Dry in segmented branches and ensure each section is thoroughly dry before moving to the next (Fig. 7.43).
- Finish the style with broad brush to ensure alignment, and finish with (optional) hairspray for long-lasting style hold (Fig. 7.44a, b).

Summary

Modern cosmetic products for hair care have evolved from basic cleansing agents into a broad plethora of agents designed to meet the needs of all women. The cosmetic industry has advanced to tailor product performance to deliver the wide range of benefits men and women want. In the development process, it takes into account regional needs and economic circumstances so that all may benefit.

Index

A
Abnormal hairs, 14–15
Accelerated weathering process, 46–47, 49
Acidic keratin proteins, 84
Acute diffuse irreversible matting, 92, 93
Acute telogen effluvium, 97
African hair shaft, flattened nature of, 34, 36
Afro-textured hair, 16
Aging, of hair, 8–9
Alopecia, 88–90
Alopecia areata, 99
Amphoteric surfactants, 107
Anagen, 6, 7
Anagen effluvium, 98, 99
Androgenetic alopecia. *See* Patterned alopecia
Anionic surfactants, 107
Antidandruff shampoos, 108
Australasian hair, 17, 18

B
Bad hair days, 31
Badly weathered hair, 46, 48
Basic keratin proteins, 84
Bird's nest hair, 58
Bleached blond hair, 22
Blond hair, 21, 22
Body hair, 1, 2
Bradford assay, 82
Brazilian keratin treatment (BKT), 67, 68, 126
Brilliantine, 110
Bubble hair, 88, 90

C
Catagen, 6
Central trichoptilosis, 88, 89
Chemical degradation, of hair, 64
Christmas tree effect, 11
Chroma reflection, 32, 36, 78
Chronic hair dehydration, 22, 23
Chronic telogen effluvium, 97, 98

Colour-treated hair, shampoos for, 109–110
Combing forces, 79
Conditioners
  brilliantine, 110
  conditioning procedure, 119–123
  conditioning variants, 110–111
  ethnic and cultural differences in, 112–114
  in ethnic usage, 111–112
  history of, 102–103
  key ingredients of, 112, 113
  mode of action, 110, 111
  oil inclusion in, 112
  silicones, 112
Conditioning (2-in-1) shampoos, 108
Cortex
  composition of, 14
  melanin granules, 14
Cross-section trichometer, 91–92
Curls and shine, 34, 36, 37
Curly hair, advantages of, 21
Cuticle, 12, 13

D
2-D electrophoresis gels, 84
Dermal papilla, 3, 4
Dermoscopy, 91
Diffuse alopecia, 88, 90
  alopecia areata, 99
  anagen effluvium, 98, 99
  patterned alopecia, 98, 99
Diffuse reflection, 32, 34

E
EDAR gene, 21
Exogen, 6
Eye-tracker technology, 52–54

F
Female pattern hair loss, 10, 86
Frictional forces, 77, 79

Frizz
    humidity-created frizz, 40–42
    loss of hair alignment, 40, 41
    manifestation of, 40, 41
    in straight hair style, 40, 41

G
Gaze plot, 53, 54
Gray hair, 22

H
Hair breakage
    in Caucasians and Asians, 89, 91
    causes of, 86
    clinical presentation
        alopecia, 88–90
        bubble hair, 88, 90
        depending on causes, 87
        depending on ethnicity, 87
        trichoclasis, 88
        trichoptilosis, 87–89
        trichorrhexis nodosa, 87–88
        trichoschisis, 88
    cross-section trichometer, 91–92
    dermoscopy, 91
    severity of, 86
    tug test, 91
Hair care and hair care products, 27
Hair-care products. *See* Conditioners; Shampoos
Hair-care product testing, 71, 72
Hair-care regimens. *See also* Conditioners; Shampoos
    history of, 103–104
    selection of
        damage repair products, 116–117
        moisture or smooth products, 115–116
        volume products, 115
Hair color, 21–22
Hair cycle
    hair growth, interruption of, 6
    kenogen, 6–8
    length of, 5
    in neonatal and early childhood period, 5
    phases of, 6–7
    schematic illustration of, 6–7
Hair damage
    causes of, 48, 49–50
    clinical signs of, 85
    global perspective, 51
    root-to-tip hair damage (*See* Root-to-tip hair damage)
    sources of, 47
    symptoms of, 85
        changes in hair colour, 94
        hair breakage, 86–92
        hair knotting, tangling, and matting, 92–94
    women's perspective, 50–51
Hair density reduction
    acute telogen effluvium, 97
    chronic telogen effluvium, 97, 98
    diffuse alopecia
        alopecia areata, 99
        anagen effluvium, 98, 99
        patterned alopecia, 98, 99
Hair diameter, 15
Hair follicle
    definition, 2
    in infancy, 2
    terminal, 3
    types of, 2–3
Hair growth
    interruption of, 6
    and nutrition, 10–11
Hair health
    assessment of hair (self/observer), 73
        breakage, 77, 79, 80
        combing forces, 79
        feel of hair, 75–76
        frictional forces, 79
        frizz assessment, 80
        instrumental methods, 76
        shine assessment, 76–78
        visual examination, 75
    connections, 104, 105
    product development for, 104
    protein changes, in hair shaft, 82–84
    single fibre mechanical properties
        tensile profile, 81
        torsion and bending, 80
        visualising damage, 81
        Young's modulus, 81
    structural property
        measures, 81–82
Hair, in time and space, 45
Hair knotting, 92–94
Hair mass, 45, 47
Hair matrix epithelium, 4
Hair phenotypes, 16
    Australasian hair, 17, 18
    Indo-European hair, 19–20
    in North and South America, 20
    oriental hair/east Asian straight hair, 17–18, 20
    sub-equatorial African hair, 16, 17
Hairspray, 127–129
Hair texture, 14
Hair thinning
    hair density, 9–10
    hair diameter, 9–10
    signs of, 9
Healthy hair signals, 31
Heat straightening, 63
Henna-coloured hair, 46, 47
Human hair
    and follicle
        definition, 2
        types of, 2–3
    function, 1
Humidity-created frizz, 40–42

Index

I
Indo-European hair, 19–20
Intensive conditioners, 111

J
Japanese straightening treatment, 126

K
Kenogen, 6–8
Keratin 31, 84

L
Lanugo hair, 11
Leave-in conditioners, 111
Localised matting, 92, 93
Lowry assay, 82
Lowry method, 55

M
Mass spectroscopy data, of soluble proteins, 82, 83
Matte effect, 34
Medulla, 14
Melanocytes, 4
Melted keratin and hair breakage, 65
Moisturising shampoos, 108

N
Natural lighter hair colors, 22
Natural shampoos, 108
Natural weathering process, 46
Nonionic surfactants, 107

O
Oriental hair/east Asian straight hair, 17–18, 20

P
Patchy alopecia, 88, 90
Patterned alopecia, 98, 99
Perhydroxyl anion (HOO^-), 65
Physical properties, of hair
  in dry conditions, 22
  elasticity, 24
  heat and humidity, 22
  porosity, 22–24
  static electricity, 24–25
Protein loss measurements, 82, 83

R
Record of the hair, 26, 47–49
Relaxer treatments, 126, 127

Rinse-out conditioners, 111, 112
Root sheath, 4
Root-to-tip hair damage
  blow drying, 64
  categories, 55, 56
  chemical treatments
    hair colouring and bleaching, 65–67
    perming, 67
    straightening and relaxing, 67–69
  cuticle degradation, 54, 55
  electron photo of, 56, 58
  environmental process, 60–63
  forms of
    cutting hair, 56
    shampooing, 58
    styling, 58
    tangling, 58–59
  heat process, 63–64
  Lowry method, 55
  minimisation, 69
  nano-structural changes, 55
  nano-to-micro-to-macro changes, 56, 57
  physical process, 59–60
  scanning electron microscope, 54
  UV exposure, 61, 63
  water hardness, 63
Root-to-tip hair health, 26–28
  absence of split ends/damaged tips, 37–40
  no breakage/strength, 43–44
  shine, 32–37
  signs of, 29, 30
  smoothness/frizz-free, 40–42
  volume, 42–43
  women's perception, 30–32

S
Scalp dermoscopy, of alopecic scalp, 89
Scalp follicles, 8
Scoring system, for hair damage, 75, 77
Seam welds, 127
Shampoos
  antidandruff, 108
  for children, 108
  for colour-treated hair, 109–110
  history of, 102
  ingredient labels, 105, 106
  key ingredients of, 107
  modern formulations, 106
  moisturising, 108
  natural, 108
  need for washing, 117–118
  polymers, 110
  qualities, 106
  shampooing procedure, 118–119
  sulphates, 107–108
  surfactant mode of action, 106–107
  washing frequency, 117, 118

Shine
- abnormal levels of, 32, 34
- chroma reflection, 32, 35
- and curls, 34, 36, 37
- diffuse reflection, 32, 34
- perception, 32, 37
- psychological aspects of, 35
- shine band, 33, 36
- specular shine, 32, 34
- styling and color, 35
- and weathering, 35–38

Special hair needs, 113
Specular reflection, 78
Specular shine, 32, 34
Split ends/damaged tips, absence of, 37–40
Spot welds, 127, 128
Stem cells, 4–5
Straight hair, advantages of, 21
Styling and hair health, 123
- guidelines for, 129–131
- hair gels/waxes/pomades, 129
- hairspray, 127–129
- mousses, 129
- straightening, 126–127
- styling problems, 124

Sub-equatorial African hair, 16, 17
Syndets, 106

T

Tangling and matting, 92–94
Teasing, 126, 127
Telogen hair, 6, 7
Terminal amino silicones (TAS), 110
Terminal hair follicle, 3
- anatomical changes of, 6
- histology and anatomy of, 5

Terminal hairs, 11, 15
Terminal hair shaft
- abnormal hairs, 14, 15
- cortex, 13–15
- cuticle, 12, 13
- description of, 11
- medulla, 14
- scanning electron microscope image of, 11

Texture, of hair, 25–26
Touch points, for hair health prediction, 71, 74
Trichoclasis, 88
Trichohyalin (TCHH), 21
Trichoptilosis, 87–89
Trichorrhexis nodosa, 87–88
Trichoschisis, 88
Tug test, 86, 91

U

Uncombable hair syndrome, 15
Unhealthy hair, psychological consequences of
- bad hair day study, 52
- hair and face as social signals, 52–55

V

Vellus hair, 12
Volume
- root-to-tip hair health, 42–43
- styling and hair health
  - blow drying, 124, 125
  - factors affecting volume, 124
  - flat/curling irons, 124–125
  - increasing hair friction, 126, 127

W

Weathering process
- accelerated weathering, 46, 49
- minimal and severe, 45, 46
- natural weathering, 46
- and shine, 35–38